# Surviving Cancer: A Formula for Hope

N.B. Singh

**DEDICATION**

To Nature,

I dedicate this book to you, the source of all life. You are my inspiration, my teacher, and my friend.

Thank you for teaching me about the beauty of the world around me. Thank you for showing me the power of the natural world. Thank you for giving me a sense of peace and tranquillity.

I promise to do my part to protect you and your many wonders. I will teach my children about the importance of conservation and sustainability. I will work to make the world a better place for all living things.

Thank you for everything, Nature.

With love,

N.B Singh

# Contents

Welcome to *Surviving Cancer: A Formula for Hope.* This book is not just a compilation of medical information and treatment protocols; it's a journey of resilience, courage, and the unwavering spirit of those who have faced the challenges of cancer.

## Why This Book?

Cancer is not just a disease; it's a life-altering experience that touches not only the patients but also their families and friends. In the face of this formidable adversary, individuals often find themselves searching for a formula—a guiding light that can illuminate the path of survival.

## The Essence of Hope

The essence of this book lies in the belief that hope is not a mere sentiment but a tangible force that can be harnessed through understanding, support, and a proactive approach to treatment. We explore the multifaceted aspects of the cancer journey, from diagnosis to survivorship, providing insights, practical advice, and a unique formula for fostering hope.

## What to Expect

In the following chapters, we delve into various dimensions of the cancer experience. From understanding the diagnosis to navigating treatment protocols, managing side effects, and embracing a holistic approach to wellness, each section is crafted to be informative, supportive, and, most importantly, filled with hope.

## A Unique Formula

At the heart of this book is the idea that hope can be expressed through a formula—an amalgamation of courage, faith, resilience, and the collective strength of a supportive community. This formula is not just a mathematical concept but a symbol of the enduring spirit that propels individuals forward on their journey.

# Join the Journey

Whether you are a patient, a caregiver, or someone seeking to understand and support those facing cancer, this book invites you to join the journey. Through narratives, practical advice, and the underlying formula for hope, we aim to empower, inspire, and foster a sense of community in the face of adversity.

**N.B. Singh**

# Chapter 1

# Introduction

## 1.1 Understanding the Diagnosis

Cancer diagnosis involves a series of critical assessments that can be simplified through practical equations and real-world insights. Let's break it down:

### 1.1.1 Cellular Abnormalities Formula

In cancer, cells undergo mutations. The probability of mutation ($P_{\text{mutation}}$) can be expressed as:

$$P_{\text{mutation}} = \frac{\text{Number of mutated cells}}{\text{Total number of cells}}$$

### 1.1.2 Genetic Profiling Equation

Understanding the genetic makeup involves analyzing various genes ($G$). The genetic profile ($GP$) can be represented as:

$$GP = \sum_{i=1}^{n} \frac{\text{Expression level of gene } i}{\text{Total number of genes}}$$

### 1.1.3 Diagnostic Sensitivity and Specificity

The accuracy of diagnostic tests is crucial. Sensitivity ($Se$) and specificity ($Sp$) are defined as:

$$Se = \frac{\text{True Positives}}{\text{True Positives} + \text{False Negatives}}$$

$$Sp = \frac{\text{True Negatives}}{\text{True Negatives} + \text{False Positives}}$$

### 1.1.4  Tumor Size Growth Rate

The growth rate ($GR$) of a tumor can be calculated over time ($t$):

$$GR = \frac{\text{Final Tumor Size} - \text{Initial Tumor Size}}{t}$$

### 1.1.5  Metastatic Potential Prediction

Assessing the risk of metastasis involves factors such as invasion ($I$) and vascularization ($V$). The metastatic potential ($MP$) can be estimated by:

$$MP = \frac{I \times V}{2}$$

### 1.1.6  Treatment Efficacy Index

Determining treatment success requires evaluating the efficacy index ($EI$):

$$EI = \frac{\text{Reduction in tumor size}}{\text{Side effects and complications}}$$

### 1.1.7  Patient Emotional Resilience

Emotional well-being is vital. The resilience index ($RI$) can be expressed as:

$$RI = \frac{\text{Positive coping mechanisms}}{\text{Negative emotional impact}}$$

Understanding these equations provides a simplified yet comprehensive view of cancer diagnosis, empowering patients and caregivers alike.

## 1.2  Emotional Impact

The emotional impact of a cancer diagnosis is profound, and understanding and managing it can be approached through both empathy and quantifiable metrics.

### 1.2.1  Emotional Distress Index

Expressing emotional distress can be quantified using the Emotional Distress Index ($EDI$):

$$EDI = \frac{\text{Intensity of distress}}{\text{Coping mechanisms employed}}$$

## 1.2.2 Calmness Quotient

Cultivating calmness is crucial. The Calmness Quotient ($CQ$) can be gauged by:

$$CQ = \frac{\text{Moments of calmness}}{\text{Total emotional upheaval}}$$

## 1.2.3 Social Support Multiplier

Social support plays a vital role. The Social Support Multiplier ($SSM$) can be calculated as:

$$SSM = \frac{\text{Number of supportive individuals}}{\text{Total social circle}}$$

## 1.2.4 Resilience Activation Formula

Activating resilience involves various factors. The Resilience Activation ($RA$) can be estimated by:

$$RA = \frac{\text{Positive mindset} + \text{Self-compassion}}{\text{Negative emotional impact}}$$

## 1.2.5 Stress Release Rate

Managing stress is key. The Stress Release Rate ($SRR$) can be represented as:

$$SRR = \frac{\text{Effective stress-relief activities}}{\text{Total stressors}}$$

## 1.2.6 Mindfulness Integration Equation

Incorporating mindfulness is beneficial. The Mindfulness Integration ($MI$) can be expressed by:

$$MI = \frac{\text{Mindful moments}}{\text{Overall thought chatter}}$$

## 1.2.7 Hopefulness Quotient

Maintaining hope is essential. The Hopefulness Quotient ($HQ$) can be measured as:

$$HQ = \frac{\text{Hopeful thoughts}}{\text{Despairing thoughts}}$$

Navigating the emotional impact of cancer involves acknowledging the complexity of emotions while quantifying the positive aspects that contribute to resilience and well-being.

## 1.3   Treatment Options

Navigating cancer treatment involves considering various options, each with its own set of factors and considerations. Let's explore them through practical insights and quantitative measures.

### 1.3.1   Treatment Effectiveness Index

Evaluating the effectiveness of a treatment can be approached using the Treatment Effectiveness Index ($TEI$):

$$TEI = \frac{\text{Reduction in tumor size}}{\text{Side effects and complications}}$$

### 1.3.2   Chemotherapy Dose Calculation

Determining the appropriate chemotherapy dose ($D$) involves patient characteristics and drug properties:

$$D = \frac{\text{Patient weight} \times \text{Drug concentration}}{\text{Body surface area}}$$

### 1.3.3   Radiation Therapy Dosage

Calculating radiation therapy dosage ($RD$) considers the targeted area and the absorbed dose:

$$RD = \frac{\text{Radiation energy absorbed}}{\text{Targeted tissue volume}}$$

### 1.3.4   Immunotherapy Response Rate

Evaluating immunotherapy success includes assessing the Response Rate ($RR$):

$$RR = \frac{\text{Number of positive responses}}{\text{Total patients treated}}$$

### 1.3.5   Surgery Success Probability

Estimating the success of a surgical procedure involves the Probability of Success ($PS$):

$$PS = \frac{\text{Number of successful surgeries}}{\text{Total surgeries performed}}$$

### 1.3.6   Treatment Affordability Index

Considering the financial aspect, the Treatment Affordability Index ($TAI$) can be calculated as:

$$TAI = \frac{\text{Treatment cost}}{\text{Patient's financial resources}}$$

### 1.3.7 Combined Modality Therapy Synergy

When employing multiple treatment modalities, the Synergy Index ($SI$) can be determined:

$$SI = \frac{\text{Combined effect of treatments}}{\text{Individual treatment effects}}$$

Navigating treatment options involves a careful balance between effectiveness, individual patient factors, and the overall impact on the quality of life.

## 1.4 Building a Support System

Creating a robust support system is essential in the journey through cancer. Let's explore practical aspects and quantify the support system's strength.

### 1.4.1 Social Network Index

Quantifying the strength of your social network can be done using the Social Network Index ($SNI$):

$$SNI = \frac{\text{Number of supportive contacts}}{\text{Total social contacts}}$$

### 1.4.2 Emotional Support Factor

Assessing the emotional support received involves the Emotional Support Factor ($ESF$):

$$ESF = \frac{\text{Number of empathetic conversations}}{\text{Total interactions}}$$

### 1.4.3 Practical Assistance Ratio

Measuring practical assistance can be done through the Practical Assistance Ratio ($PAR$):

$$PAR = \frac{\text{Number of helpful actions}}{\text{Total requests for assistance}}$$

### 1.4.4 Communication Openness Score

Encouraging open communication is crucial. The Communication Openness Score ($COS$) can be determined as:

$$COS = \frac{\text{Frequency of open conversations}}{\text{Total communication instances}}$$

### 1.4.5 Reliability Coefficient

Reliability in support is vital. The Reliability Coefficient ($RC$) can be calculated using:

$$RC = \frac{\text{Dependability of support}}{\text{Instances of unmet expectations}}$$

### 1.4.6 Financial Support Index

Incorporating financial support, the Financial Support Index ($FSI$) is defined as:

$$FSI = \frac{\text{Financial assistance received}}{\text{Total financial burden}}$$

### 1.4.7 Support Diversity Quotient

A diverse support system is valuable. The Support Diversity Quotient ($SDQ$) can be expressed as:

$$SDQ = \frac{\text{Number of different support sources}}{\text{Total support providers}}$$

Building a support system involves both qualitative and quantitative aspects, ensuring a well-rounded network to navigate the challenges of cancer.

## 1.5 Mind-Body Connection

Understanding the intricate link between the mind and body is crucial for holistic well-being. Let's explore this connection through practical insights and quantifiable measures.

### 1.5.1 Stress Reduction Equation

Reducing stress is essential. The Stress Reduction Equation ($SR$) is given by:

$$SR = \frac{\text{Effective stress-relief activities}}{\text{Total stressors}}$$

### 1.5.2 Mindfulness Integration Index

Incorporating mindfulness is beneficial. The Mindfulness Integration Index ($MII$) is expressed as:

$$MII = \frac{\text{Moments of mindfulness}}{\text{Overall thought activity}}$$

### 1.5.3 Emotional Resilience Ratio

Building emotional resilience involves the Emotional Resilience Ratio ($ERR$):

$$ERR = \frac{\text{Positive coping mechanisms}}{\text{Negative emotional impact}}$$

### 1.5.4 Physical Activity Relaxation Quotient

The relaxation gained from physical activity can be measured by the Physical Activity Relaxation Quotient ($PARQ$):

$$PARQ = \frac{\text{Relaxation after exercise}}{\text{Intensity and duration of exercise}}$$

### 1.5.5 Neurotransmitter Harmony Index

Balancing neurotransmitters is key. The Neurotransmitter Harmony Index ($NHI$) can be determined as:

$$NHI = \frac{\text{Balanced neurotransmitter levels}}{\text{Neurotransmitter fluctuations}}$$

### 1.5.6 Sleep Quality Score

Quality sleep is vital. The Sleep Quality Score ($SQS$) can be represented as:

$$SQS = \frac{\text{Restorative sleep duration}}{\text{Total time in bed}}$$

### 1.5.7 Positive Affirmation Boost Factor

Utilizing positive affirmations contributes to well-being. The Positive Affirmation Boost Factor ($PABF$) is defined by:

$$PABF = \frac{\text{Positive affirmations internalized}}{\text{Negative self-talk instances}}$$

Exploring the mind-body connection involves quantifiable factors that contribute to overall health and resilience.

## 1.6 Hope as a Catalyst

Hope serves as a powerful catalyst in the face of challenges. Let's explore the dynamics of hope through practical insights and quantifiable measures.

### 1.6.1  Hopefulness Quotient

Maintaining hope can be measured by the Hopefulness Quotient ($HQ$):

$$HQ = \frac{\text{Hopeful thoughts}}{\text{Despairing thoughts}}$$

### 1.6.2  Positive Visualization Impact

Visualizing positive outcomes impacts well-being. The Positive Visualization Impact ($PVI$) is given by:

$$PVI = \frac{\text{Number of positive visualizations}}{\text{Total visualizations}}$$

### 1.6.3  Hope Resilience Index

Building resilience through hope involves the Hope Resilience Index ($HRI$):

$$HRI = \frac{\text{Positive coping mechanisms}}{\text{Negative emotional impact}}$$

### 1.6.4  Future Expectation Equation

Expecting positive outcomes contributes to hope. The Future Expectation Equation ($FEQ$) is expressed as:

$$FEQ = \frac{\text{Expectation of positive events}}{\text{Expectation of negative events}}$$

### 1.6.5  Hopeful Goal Attainment Ratio

Setting and achieving hopeful goals is crucial. The Hopeful Goal Attainment Ratio ($HGAR$) is calculated by:

$$HGAR = \frac{\text{Achieved hopeful goals}}{\text{Total set hopeful goals}}$$

### 1.6.6  Optimism Resonance Factor

Optimism resonates with hope. The Optimism Resonance Factor ($ORF$) can be determined as:

$$ORF = \frac{\text{Optimistic outlook instances}}{\text{Pessimistic outlook instances}}$$

### 1.6.7 Hope Sustenance Coefficient

Sustaining hope involves the Hope Sustenance Coefficient ($HSC$):

$$HSC = \frac{\text{Continuous hopeful thoughts}}{\text{Interruptions by despairing thoughts}}$$

Exploring hope as a catalyst involves understanding its quantifiable impact on mindset and resilience.

## 1.7 Facing the Unknown

Navigating uncertainty requires a blend of practical insights and quantifiable measures. Let's delve into facing the unknown with real-world considerations.

### 1.7.1 Risk Tolerance Index

Facing the unknown involves assessing risk tolerance through the Risk Tolerance Index ($RTI$):

$$RTI = \frac{\text{Comfort with uncertainty}}{\text{Discomfort with uncertainty}}$$

### 1.7.2 Adaptability Quotient

Adapting to the unknown is crucial. The Adaptability Quotient ($AQ$) is given by:

$$AQ = \frac{\text{Successful adaptations}}{\text{Instances of resistance to change}}$$

### 1.7.3 Information Absorption Rate

Gaining insights helps in facing uncertainty. The Information Absorption Rate ($IAR$) is expressed as:

$$IAR = \frac{\text{Effective information absorption}}{\text{Total information encountered}}$$

### 1.7.4 Decision Confidence Ratio

Making decisions in uncertainty involves the Decision Confidence Ratio ($DCR$):

$$DCR = \frac{\text{Confident decisions made}}{\text{Instances of decision hesitation}}$$

### 1.7.5    Ambiguity Resilience Coefficient

Building resilience to ambiguity is essential. The Ambiguity Resilience Coefficient ($ARC$) can be calculated as:

$$ARC = \frac{\text{Resilience in ambiguous situations}}{\text{Instances of feeling overwhelmed}}$$

### 1.7.6    Uncertainty Navigation Index

Effectively navigating uncertainty is measured by the Uncertainty Navigation Index ($UNI$):

$$UNI = \frac{\text{Successfully navigated uncertain situations}}{\text{Instances of uncertainty-induced stress}}$$

### 1.7.7    Fear Management Equation

Facing the unknown involves managing fear. The Fear Management Equation ($FME$) is expressed by:

$$FME = \frac{\text{Effective fear coping mechanisms}}{\text{Instances of fear paralysis}}$$

Confronting the unknown involves understanding one's capacity for adaptation, resilience, and decision-making in the face of uncertainty.

# Chapter 2

# The Journey Begins

## 2.1 First Steps to Recovery

Embarking on the path to recovery involves practical steps and quantifiable measures to initiate healing.

### 2.1.1 Physical Activity Kickstart

Initiate physical activity with the Exercise Ignition Formula ($EIF$):

$$EIF = \frac{\text{Motivation to Exercise}}{\text{Barriers to Exercise}}$$

### 2.1.2 Nutritional Reboot

Rejuvenate nutrition with the Nutrient Boost Quotient ($NBQ$):

$$NBQ = \frac{\text{Nutrient-rich foods consumed}}{\text{Processed foods intake}}$$

### 2.1.3 Sleep Restoration Factor

Restore sleep with the Sleep Quality Recharge ($SQR$):

$$SQR = \frac{\text{Restorative sleep hours}}{\text{Total time in bed}}$$

### 2.1.4   Stress Relief Catalyst

Kickstart stress relief with the Stress Dissipation Ratio ($SDR$):

$$SDR = \frac{\text{Effective stress-relief activities}}{\text{Total stressors}}$$

### 2.1.5   Mindfulness Commencement

Commence mindfulness practices with the Mindful Moments Index ($MMI$):

$$MMI = \frac{\text{Moments of mindfulness}}{\text{Overall thought activity}}$$

### 2.1.6   Support System Activation

Activate your support system using the Support Engagement Index ($SEI$):

$$SEI = \frac{\text{Active support interactions}}{\text{Total support network}}$$

### 2.1.7   Hopefulness Kickoff

Initiate hope with the Hope Infusion Quotient ($HIQ$):

$$HIQ = \frac{\text{Hopeful thoughts}}{\text{Despairing thoughts}}$$

Taking these initial steps with measurable approaches sets the foundation for a strong and purposeful recovery journey.

## 2.2   Navigating Treatment Protocols

Navigating treatment involves practical steps and quantifiable measures to optimize the healing process.

### 2.2.1   Treatment Effectiveness Gauge

Evaluate treatment effectiveness with the Treatment Efficacy Score ($TES$):

$$TES = \frac{\text{Positive outcomes achieved}}{\text{Total treatment interventions}}$$

### 2.2.2 Chemotherapy Personalization

Tailor chemotherapy using the Personalized Dose Equation ($PDE$):

$$PDE = \frac{\text{Patient weight} \times \text{Drug concentration}}{\text{Body surface area}}$$

### 2.2.3 Radiation Precision Index

Optimize radiation therapy with the Targeted Dose Precision ($TDP$):

$$TDP = \frac{\text{Radiation energy absorbed}}{\text{Targeted tissue volume}}$$

### 2.2.4 Immunotherapy Response Monitor

Track immunotherapy response using the Immunotherapy Response Index ($IRI$):

$$IRI = \frac{\text{Positive responses observed}}{\text{Total patients treated}}$$

### 2.2.5 Surgery Success Predictor

Predict surgery success with the Surgical Outcome Probability ($SOP$):

$$SOP = \frac{\text{Successful surgeries performed}}{\text{Total surgeries conducted}}$$

### 2.2.6 Financial Impact Assessment

Assess the financial impact with the Cost-Benefit Index ($CBI$):

$$CBI = \frac{\text{Treatment benefits}}{\text{Financial burden incurred}}$$

### 2.2.7 Combined Modality Synergy

Enhance treatment synergy with the Combined Modality Impact ($CMI$):

$$CMI = \frac{\text{Collective treatment effectiveness}}{\text{Individual treatment impacts}}$$

Navigating treatment protocols involves optimizing interventions with measurable outcomes for a purposeful journey.

## 2.3   Nutritional Support

Optimizing nutrition is a vital part of the healing journey, blending practical insights with quantifiable measures.

### 2.3.1   Nutrient Density Gauge

Evaluate nutrient intake with the Nutrient Density Score ($NDS$):

$$NDS = \frac{\text{Essential nutrients consumed}}{\text{Total calorie intake}}$$

### 2.3.2   Protein Power Equation

Boost protein intake with the Protein Efficacy Formula ($PEF$):

$$PEF = \frac{\text{Protein intake}}{\text{Body weight}}$$

### 2.3.3   Micronutrient Harmony

Maintain micronutrient balance with the Micronutrient Ratio ($MR$):

$$MR = \frac{\text{Individual micronutrient levels}}{\text{Recommended daily intake}}$$

### 2.3.4   Hydration Quotient

Ensure hydration with the Hydration Index ($HI$):

$$HI = \frac{\text{Fluid intake}}{\text{Body weight}}$$

### 2.3.5   Gut Health Index

Support gut health with the Gut Microbiota Balance ($GMB$):

$$GMB = \frac{\text{Beneficial bacteria count}}{\text{Total gut microbiota}}$$

### 2.3.6   Antioxidant Boost Factor

Enhance antioxidants with the Antioxidant Amplification ($AA$):

$$AA = \frac{\text{Antioxidant-rich foods consumed}}{\text{Total daily antioxidants needed}}$$

### 2.3.7 Energy Balance Equation

Maintain energy balance with the Caloric Equilibrium ($CE$):

$$CE = \frac{\text{Calories consumed}}{\text{Calories expended}}$$

Nutritional support involves a balanced and personalized approach, integrating essential nutrients for a resilient recovery journey.

## 2.4 Managing Side Effects

Effectively addressing side effects involves practical steps and quantifiable measures for a smoother journey.

### 2.4.1 Symptom Severity Scale

Quantify symptom severity using the Symptom Impact Score ($SIS$):

$$SIS = \frac{\text{Impact of symptoms on daily life}}{\text{Total number of symptoms}}$$

### 2.4.2 Medication Tolerance Index

Assess medication tolerance with the Medication Compatibility Ratio ($MCR$):

$$MCR = \frac{\text{Comfort with medications}}{\text{Discomfort with medications}}$$

### 2.4.3 Fatigue Resilience Factor

Build resilience against fatigue using the Fatigue Management Coefficient ($FMC$):

$$FMC = \frac{\text{Effective fatigue coping mechanisms}}{\text{Instances of overwhelming fatigue}}$$

### 2.4.4 Nausea Repellent Equation

Combat nausea with the Anti-Nausea Index ($ANI$):

$$ANI = \frac{\text{Effectiveness of anti-nausea strategies}}{\text{Frequency of nausea episodes}}$$

### 2.4.5 Pain Tolerance Quotient

Assess pain tolerance with the Pain Resilience Scale ($PRS$):

$$PRS = \frac{\text{Ability to cope with pain}}{\text{Intensity and duration of pain}}$$

### 2.4.6 Cognitive Clarity Index

Maintain cognitive clarity with the Mental Sharpness Quotient ($MSQ$):

$$MSQ = \frac{\text{Clarity of thought}}{\text{Instances of mental fog}}$$

### 2.4.7 Emotional Stability Ratio

Stabilize emotions with the Emotional Resilience Coefficient ($ERC$):

$$ERC = \frac{\text{Resilience against emotional fluctuations}}{\text{Intensity of emotional distress}}$$

Managing side effects involves proactive measures and personalized strategies to enhance overall well-being during the journey.

## 2.5 Coping Strategies

Navigating challenges requires practical coping strategies and quantifiable measures for resilience.

### 2.5.1 Stress Reduction Formula

Reduce stress with the Stress Dissipation Ratio ($SDR$):

$$SDR = \frac{\text{Effective stress-relief activities}}{\text{Total stressors}}$$

### 2.5.2 Mindfulness Integration Index

Incorporate mindfulness using the Mindfulness Adoption Quotient ($MAQ$):

$$MAQ = \frac{\text{Moments of mindfulness}}{\text{Overall thought activity}}$$

### 2.5.3 Emotional Resilience Coefficient

Build emotional resilience with the Emotional Stability Index ($ESI$):

$$ESI = \frac{\text{Positive coping mechanisms}}{\text{Negative emotional impact}}$$

### 2.5.4 Social Connection Quotient

Enhance social connections with the Social Engagement Ratio ($SER$):

$$SER = \frac{\text{Quality interactions}}{\text{Total social interactions}}$$

### 2.5.5 Positive Affirmation Boost

Boost positivity with the Affirmation Impact Factor ($AIF$):

$$AIF = \frac{\text{Positive affirmations internalized}}{\text{Instances of negative self-talk}}$$

### 2.5.6 Humor Resilience Index

Utilize humor for resilience with the Humor Uplift Quotient ($HUQ$):

$$HUQ = \frac{\text{Moments of laughter}}{\text{Total challenging situations}}$$

### 2.5.7 Adaptability Quotient

Enhance adaptability using the Adaptation Readiness Score ($ARS$):

$$ARS = \frac{\text{Successful adaptations}}{\text{Instances of resistance to change}}$$

Coping strategies involve a blend of mindfulness, social connection, and positive reinforcement, creating a foundation for resilience during the journey.

## 2.6 Empowering Through Education

Empowering through education involves practical insights and quantifiable measures to enhance understanding.

### 2.6.1   Knowledge Retention Quotient

Boost knowledge retention with the Learning Efficiency Score ($LES$):

$$LES = \frac{\text{Effective learning instances}}{\text{Total learning opportunities}}$$

### 2.6.2   Information Application Index

Apply information effectively using the Application Proficiency Quotient ($APQ$):

$$APQ = \frac{\text{Applied knowledge instances}}{\text{Total knowledge acquired}}$$

### 2.6.3   Resource Utilization Equation

Optimize resource use with the Resource Efficiency Formula ($REF$):

$$REF = \frac{\text{Effective utilization of resources}}{\text{Total available resources}}$$

### 2.6.4   Decision-making Competence

Enhance decision-making with the Decision Competence Index ($DCI$):

$$DCI = \frac{\text{Quality decisions made}}{\text{Instances of decision hesitation}}$$

### 2.6.5   Risk Understanding Ratio

Comprehend risks effectively with the Risk Perception Quotient ($RPQ$):

$$RPQ = \frac{\text{Accurate risk assessments}}{\text{Instances of risk misjudgment}}$$

### 2.6.6   Communication Clarity Factor

Improve communication with the Clarity in Expression Score ($CES$):

$$CES = \frac{\text{Clear communication instances}}{\text{Total communication interactions}}$$

### 2.6.7   Skill Acquisition Accelerator

Accelerate skill acquisition with the Skill Mastery Rate ($SMR$):

$$SMR = \frac{\text{Mastery of new skills}}{\text{Total skills attempted}}$$

Empowering through education involves maximizing learning potential, applying knowledge effectively, and making informed decisions on the journey.

## 2.7 Finding Strength in Community

Harnessing strength from community involves practical insights and quantifiable measures for mutual support.

### 2.7.1 Support Density Index

Measure support density with the Supportive Connections Ratio ($SCR$):

$$SCR = \frac{\text{Supportive relationships}}{\text{Total relationships}}$$

### 2.7.2 Empathy Amplification

Amplify empathy with the Empathy Impact Factor ($EIF$):

$$EIF = \frac{\text{Empathetic actions taken}}{\text{Total opportunities for empathy}}$$

### 2.7.3 Collective Resilience Quotient

Quantify collective resilience with the Community Resilience Index ($CRI$):

$$CRI = \frac{\text{Community's positive response instances}}{\text{Challenges faced by the community}}$$

### 2.7.4 Collaborative Strength Equation

Enhance collaborative strength with the Collaborative Power Factor ($CPF$):

$$CPF = \frac{\text{Collaborative efforts' impact}}{\text{Total collaborative endeavors}}$$

### 2.7.5 Shared Goal Attainment

Achieve shared goals with the Communal Success Ratio ($CSR$):

$$CSR = \frac{\text{Achieved communal goals}}{\text{Total communal goals set}}$$

### 2.7.6 Unified Support Amplifier

Amplify unified support with the Support Unity Multiplier ($SUM$):

$$SUM = \frac{\text{Unified support instances}}{\text{Total support interactions}}$$

### 2.7.7 Collective Hopefulness Index

Quantify collective hope with the Community Hopefulness Quotient ($CHQ$):

$$CHQ = \frac{\text{Collective hopeful thoughts}}{\text{Collective despairing thoughts}}$$

Finding strength in community involves fostering supportive relationships, collaborative efforts, and a shared sense of hope on the journey.

# Chapter 3

# Resilience in Treatment

## 3.1 Chemotherapy Insights

Navigating chemotherapy involves practical insights and quantifiable measures for resilience.

### 3.1.1 Tumor Response Equation

Assess tumor response with the Tumor Response Index ($TRI$):

$$TRI = \frac{\text{Reduction in tumor size}}{\text{Chemotherapy sessions}}$$

### 3.1.2 Chemotherapy Dosage Optimization

Optimize chemotherapy dosage with the Dosage Adjustment Formula ($DAF$):

$$DAF = \frac{\text{Patient weight} \times \text{Drug concentration}}{\text{Body surface area}}$$

### 3.1.3 Side Effect Mitigation

Mitigate side effects with the Side Effect Management Quotient ($SEM$):

$$SEM = \frac{\text{Effective side effect management}}{\text{Total side effects experienced}}$$

### 3.1.4 Treatment Affordability Index

Consider treatment affordability with the Chemotherapy Affordability Score ($CAS$):

$$CAS = \frac{\text{Treatment cost}}{\text{Patient's financial resources}}$$

### 3.1.5 Chemotherapy Resilience Coefficient

Build resilience during chemotherapy with the Chemo Resilience Factor ($CRF$):

$$CRF = \frac{\text{Resilience against treatment-related stress}}{\text{Instances of treatment-related distress}}$$

### 3.1.6 Chemotherapy Response Rate

Evaluate chemotherapy response with the Chemotherapy Effectiveness Ratio ($CER$):

$$CER = \frac{\text{Positive responses observed}}{\text{Total chemotherapy sessions}}$$

### 3.1.7 Molecular Targeting Precision

Enhance precision with Molecular Targeting Efficiency ($MTE$):

$$MTE = \frac{\text{Effectiveness of molecular targeting agents}}{\text{Total molecular targeting interventions}}$$

Chemotherapy insights involve optimizing dosage, managing side effects, and building resilience for a purposeful treatment journey.

## 3.2 Radiation Therapy Essentials

Mastering radiation therapy involves practical insights and quantifiable measures for resilience.

### 3.2.1 Targeted Dose Precision

Optimize dose precision with the Targeted Dose Efficiency ($TDE$):

$$TDE = \frac{\text{Radiation energy absorbed}}{\text{Targeted tissue volume}}$$

### 3.2.2  Radiation Resilience Index

Build resilience during radiation therapy with the Radiation Resilience Quotient ($RRQ$):

$$RRQ = \frac{\text{Resilience against radiation-induced stress}}{\text{Instances of radiation-related distress}}$$

### 3.2.3  Side Effect Mitigation

Mitigate side effects with the Radiation Side Effect Management ($RSEM$):

$$RSEM = \frac{\text{Effective side effect management}}{\text{Total side effects experienced}}$$

### 3.2.4  Treatment Affordability Ratio

Consider treatment affordability with the Radiation Affordability Index ($RAI$):

$$RAI = \frac{\text{Treatment cost}}{\text{Patient's financial resources}}$$

### 3.2.5  Radiation Response Rate

Evaluate radiation response with the Radiation Effectiveness Quotient ($REQ$):

$$REQ = \frac{\text{Positive responses observed}}{\text{Total radiation sessions}}$$

### 3.2.6  Dose Escalation Equation

Optimize treatment intensity with the Dose Escalation Formula ($DEF$):

$$DEF = \frac{\text{Increased radiation dose}}{\text{Total treatment sessions}}$$

### 3.2.7  Molecular Targeting Precision

Enhance precision with Molecular Targeting Efficiency ($MTE$):

$$MTE = \frac{\text{Effectiveness of molecular targeting agents}}{\text{Total molecular targeting interventions}}$$

Radiation therapy essentials involve precise targeting, resilience-building, and effective side effect management for a purposeful treatment journey.

## 3.3   Surgical Approaches

Navigating surgery involves practical insights and quantifiable measures for resilience.

### 3.3.1   Surgery Success Index

Assess surgery success with the Surgical Outcome Quotient ($SOQ$):

$$SOQ = \frac{\text{Successful surgeries performed}}{\text{Total surgeries conducted}}$$

### 3.3.2   Anesthesia Tolerance Ratio

Evaluate anesthesia tolerance with the Anesthesia Compatibility Factor ($ACF$):

$$ACF = \frac{\text{Tolerance to anesthesia}}{\text{Instances of discomfort with anesthesia}}$$

### 3.3.3   Recovery Acceleration

Accelerate recovery with the Post-Surgery Recovery Rate ($PSRR$):

$$PSRR = \frac{\text{Speed of recovery}}{\text{Anticipated recovery time}}$$

### 3.3.4   Postoperative Pain Management

Manage postoperative pain with the Pain Relief Efficiency ($PRE$):

$$PRE = \frac{\text{Effective pain relief interventions}}{\text{Total postoperative pain episodes}}$$

### 3.3.5   Wound Healing Quotient

Enhance wound healing with the Wound Recovery Index ($WRI$):

$$WRI = \frac{\text{Speed of wound healing}}{\text{Expected healing time}}$$

### 3.3.6   Complication Prevention Score

Prevent complications with the Surgery Complication Prevention ($SCP$):

$$SCP = \frac{\text{Preventative measures taken}}{\text{Instances of postoperative complications}}$$

### 3.3.7  Surgery Affordability Index

Consider surgery affordability with the Surgical Affordability Score ($SAS$):

$$SAS = \frac{\text{Surgery cost}}{\text{Patient's financial resources}}$$

Surgical approaches involve optimizing success, managing recovery, and ensuring a resilient journey through and after the procedure.

## 3.4  Complementary Therapies

Complementary therapies involve practical insights and quantifiable measures for resilience.

### 3.4.1  Mindfulness Integration

Integrate mindfulness with the Mindful Practice Quotient ($MPQ$):

$$MPQ = \frac{\text{Time spent in mindful practices}}{\text{Total daily activities}}$$

### 3.4.2  Herbal Support Synergy

Leverage herbal support with the Herbal Complementarity Index ($HCI$):

$$HCI = \frac{\text{Effectiveness of herbal supplements}}{\text{Total complementary interventions}}$$

### 3.4.3  Acupuncture Resilience Factor

Enhance resilience with acupuncture using the Acupuncture Impact Score ($AIS$):

$$AIS = \frac{\text{Positive effects of acupuncture}}{\text{Total acupuncture sessions}}$$

### 3.4.4  Yoga Flexibility Ratio

Improve flexibility with yoga using the Flexibility Enhancement Quotient ($FEQ$):

$$FEQ = \frac{\text{Flexibility gains}}{\text{Total yoga sessions}}$$

### 3.4.5   Massage Therapy Relaxation

Promote relaxation with massage therapy using the Relaxation Induction Index ($RII$):

$$RII = \frac{\text{Relaxation induced by massage}}{\text{Total massage sessions}}$$

### 3.4.6   Art Therapy Expression

Express through art therapy with the Artistic Expression Score ($AES$):

$$AES = \frac{\text{Positive emotional expression}}{\text{Total art therapy sessions}}$$

### 3.4.7   Music Therapy Harmony

Find harmony with music therapy through the Harmonious Resonance Quotient ($HRQ$):

$$HRQ = \frac{\text{Harmony achieved through music}}{\text{Total music therapy sessions}}$$

Complementary therapies involve integrating practices that enhance well-being, fostering resilience alongside conventional treatments.


## 3.5   Mindfulness Practices

Embracing mindfulness involves practical insights and quantifiable measures for resilience.


### 3.5.1   Mindful Breath Ratio

Engage in mindful breathing with the Breath Awareness Quotient ($BAQ$):

$$BAQ = \frac{\text{Mindful breaths taken}}{\text{Total breaths in a minute}}$$

### 3.5.2   Present Moment Index

Cultivate presence with the Present-Moment Awareness Score ($PMAS$):

$$PMAS = \frac{\text{Moments fully present}}{\text{Total waking moments}}$$

### 3.5.3  Mindful Walking Efficiency

Optimize mindful walking with the Walk Awareness Index ($WAI$):

$$WAI = \frac{\text{Mindful steps taken}}{\text{Total steps during walking}}$$

### 3.5.4  Body Scan Effectiveness

Enhance body scan mindfulness with the Body Awareness Quotient ($BAQ$):

$$BAQ = \frac{\text{Effective body scan moments}}{\text{Total body scan sessions}}$$

### 3.5.5  Mindful Eating Awareness

Improve mindful eating with the Nutritional Mindfulness Score ($NMS$):

$$NMS = \frac{\text{Mindful bites taken}}{\text{Total bites during a meal}}$$

### 3.5.6  Mindful Sleep Quality

Promote mindful sleep with the Sleep Awareness Ratio ($SAR$):

$$SAR = \frac{\text{Mindful moments before sleep}}{\text{Total pre-sleep moments}}$$

### 3.5.7  Mindful Stress Response

Manage stress mindfully with the Mindful Stress Resilience ($MSR$):

$$MSR = \frac{\text{Effective stress responses}}{\text{Total stress-triggered moments}}$$

Mindfulness practices involve integrating awareness into daily activities, fostering resilience and well-being throughout the treatment journey.

## 3.6  Family Dynamics During Treatment

Navigating family dynamics involves practical insights and quantifiable measures for resilience.

### 3.6.1   Family Support Quotient

Measure family support with the Family Support Index ($FSI$):

$$FSI = \frac{\text{Effective family support instances}}{\text{Total support opportunities}}$$

### 3.6.2   Communication Harmony

Foster communication harmony with the Communication Synchronization ($CS$):

$$CS = \frac{\text{Smooth communication instances}}{\text{Total communication interactions}}$$

### 3.6.3   Emotional Resilience Nexus

Build emotional resilience within the family using the Emotional Resilience Coefficient ($ERC$):

$$ERC = \frac{\text{Family's resilience against emotional fluctuations}}{\text{Intensity of emotional distress}}$$

### 3.6.4   Shared Responsibility Ratio

Allocate responsibilities effectively with the Responsibility Distribution Index ($RDI$):

$$RDI = \frac{\text{Fair distribution of responsibilities}}{\text{Instances of role conflict}}$$

### 3.6.5   Family Well-being Quotient

Assess family well-being with the Family Harmony Score ($FHS$):

$$FHS = \frac{\text{Positive family interactions}}{\text{Total family interactions}}$$

### 3.6.6   Adaptability Resilience

Enhance adaptability within the family using the Family Adaptation Quotient ($FAQ$):

$$FAQ = \frac{\text{Successful family adaptations}}{\text{Instances of resistance to change}}$$

### 3.6.7   Collective Hopefulness Index

Quantify collective hope with the Family Hopefulness Quotient ($FHQ$):

$$FHQ = \frac{\text{Collective hopeful thoughts}}{\text{Collective despairing thoughts}}$$

Family dynamics during treatment involve fostering support, communication, and shared resilience for a purposeful journey.

## 3.7 Monitoring Your Progress

Monitoring progress involves practical insights and quantifiable measures for resilience.

### 3.7.1 Resilience Reflection Score

Reflect on resilience with the Resilience Reflection Index ($RRI$):

$$RRI = \frac{\text{Moments of self-reflection on resilience}}{\text{Total self-reflection opportunities}}$$

### 3.7.2 Treatment Milestone Tracker

Track treatment milestones with the Milestone Achievement Ratio ($MAR$):

$$MAR = \frac{\text{Achieved treatment milestones}}{\text{Total treatment milestones set}}$$

### 3.7.3 Well-being Check-in

Check well-being regularly with the Well-being Assessment Frequency ($WAF$):

$$WAF = \frac{\text{Well-being assessments performed}}{\text{Total well-being check-ins}}$$

### 3.7.4 Mindfulness Progress Gauge

Gauge mindfulness progress with the Mindful Growth Index ($MGI$):

$$MGI = \frac{\text{Mindfulness improvement instances}}{\text{Total mindfulness practice sessions}}$$

### 3.7.5 Resilience Journaling

Capture resilience moments with the Resilience Journaling Efficiency ($RJE$):

$$RJE = \frac{\text{Positive reflections recorded}}{\text{Total journaling sessions}}$$

### 3.7.6  Health Metrics Mastery

Master health metrics with the Health Data Competence ($HDC$):

$$HDC = \frac{\text{Effective interpretation of health metrics}}{\text{Total health data assessments}}$$

### 3.7.7  Positive Affirmation Reinforcement

Reinforce positivity with the Affirmation Reinforcement Quotient ($ARQ$):

$$ARQ = \frac{\text{Positive affirmations internalized}}{\text{Instances of negative self-talk}}$$

Monitoring progress involves consistent self-reflection and quantifiable measures, fostering resilience on the treatment journey.

# Chapter 4

# Healing Mind and Body

## 4.1 Holistic Wellness

Embracing holistic wellness involves practical insights and quantifiable measures for a balanced mind and body.

### 4.1.1 Wellness Equation

Balance wellness with the Holistic Wellness Quotient ($HWQ$):

$$HWQ = \frac{\text{Mental well-being} + \text{Physical well-being}}{2}$$

### 4.1.2 Nutrient-Packed Diet

Fuel the body with the Nutrient Density Score ($NDS$):

$$NDS = \frac{\text{Essential nutrients consumed}}{\text{Total calorie intake}}$$

### 4.1.3 Mindfulness Integration

Infuse mindfulness into daily life with the Mindful Living Index ($MLI$):

$$MLI = \frac{\text{Moments lived mindfully}}{\text{Total waking moments}}$$

### 4.1.4 Physical Activity Optimization

Optimize physical activity with the Exercise Efficiency Ratio ($EER$):

$$EER = \frac{\text{Effective exercise sessions}}{\text{Total exercise attempts}}$$

### 4.1.5 Quality Sleep Attainment

Achieve quality sleep with the Sleep Quality Index ($SQI$):

$$SQI = \frac{\text{Restful sleep instances}}{\text{Total sleep opportunities}}$$

### 4.1.6 Stress Resilience Formula

Build resilience against stress with the Stress Resilience Coefficient ($SRC$):

$$SRC = \frac{\text{Positive stress coping mechanisms}}{\text{Negative impact of stress}}$$

### 4.1.7 Social Connection Synergy

Foster social connections with the Social Engagement Ratio ($SER$):

$$SER = \frac{\text{Quality interactions}}{\text{Total social interactions}}$$

Holistic wellness involves a harmonious blend of mental and physical well-being, fostering a balanced and resilient life.

## 4.2 Embracing a Healthy Lifestyle

Adopting a healthy lifestyle involves practical insights and quantifiable measures for overall well-being.

### 4.2.1 Balanced Diet Harmony

Achieve diet balance with the Nutrient Harmony Index ($NHI$):

$$NHI = \frac{\text{Macro and micronutrient balance}}{\text{Total daily nutrients}}$$

### 4.2.2   Physical Activity Integration

Incorporate physical activity with the Activity Inclusion Ratio ($AIR$):

$$AIR = \frac{\text{Physical activities included in daily routine}}{\text{Total daily activities}}$$

### 4.2.3   Hydration Quotient

Ensure hydration with the Hydration Index ($HI$):

$$HI = \frac{\text{Fluid intake}}{\text{Body weight}}$$

### 4.2.4   Sleep Quality Index

Optimize sleep quality with the Sleep Quality Index ($SQI$):

$$SQI = \frac{\text{Restful sleep instances}}{\text{Total sleep opportunities}}$$

### 4.2.5   Stress Management Equation

Manage stress with the Stress Coping Efficiency ($SCE$):

$$SCE = \frac{\text{Effective stress coping mechanisms}}{\text{Total stress-triggered moments}}$$

### 4.2.6   Social Connection Synergy

Foster social connections with the Social Engagement Ratio ($SER$):

$$SER = \frac{\text{Quality interactions}}{\text{Total social interactions}}$$

### 4.2.7   Mindful Living Index

Infuse mindfulness into daily life with the Mindful Living Index ($MLI$):

$$MLI = \frac{\text{Moments lived mindfully}}{\text{Total waking moments}}$$

Embracing a healthy lifestyle involves creating a balance in diet, physical activity, sleep, stress management, social connections, and mindful living for a resilient and vibrant life.

## 4.3 Mind-Body Harmony

Achieving mind-body harmony involves practical insights and quantifiable measures for a synchronized and balanced existence.

### 4.3.1 Stress-Busting Breath Ratio

Calm the mind with the Breath Relaxation Quotient ($BRQ$):

$$BRQ = \frac{\text{Mindful breaths taken}}{\text{Total breaths in a minute}}$$

### 4.3.2 Emotional Resilience Index

Strengthen emotional resilience with the Emotion Resilience Coefficient ($ERC$):

$$ERC = \frac{\text{Positive emotional coping mechanisms}}{\text{Negative emotional impact}}$$

### 4.3.3 Mental Clarity Quotient

Enhance mental clarity with the Mind Sharpness Index ($MSI$):

$$MSI = \frac{\text{Clarity of thought}}{\text{Instances of mental fog}}$$

### 4.3.4 Nutrient Harmony Formula

Support the body with the Nutrient Equilibrium Index ($NEI$):

$$NEI = \frac{\text{Balanced nutrient intake}}{\text{Total daily nutritional needs}}$$

### 4.3.5 Physical-Emotional Synchronization

Synchronize physical and emotional well-being with the Wellness Alignment Ratio ($WAR$):

$$WAR = \frac{\text{Physical well-being score} + \text{Emotional well-being score}}{2}$$

### 4.3.6 Mindful Movement Efficiency

Optimize mindful movement with the Movement Awareness Quotient ($MAQ$):

$$MAQ = \frac{\text{Mindful movements}}{\text{Total movements during a day}}$$

### 4.3.7 Positive Affirmation Boost

Uplift positivity with the Affirmation Impact Factor ($AIF$):

$$AIF = \frac{\text{Positive affirmations internalized}}{\text{Instances of negative self-talk}}$$

Mind-body harmony involves synchronized well-being, fostering balance and resilience in everyday life.

## 4.4 Spiritual Resilience

Nurturing spiritual resilience involves practical insights and quantifiable measures for a resilient and harmonious inner self.

### 4.4.1 Mindful Reflection Quotient

Cultivate spiritual resilience with the Reflection Awareness Index ($RAI$):

$$RAI = \frac{\text{Mindful moments of self-reflection}}{\text{Total waking moments}}$$

### 4.4.2 Gratitude Amplification

Amplify gratitude with the Gratitude Expansion Ratio ($GER$):

$$GER = \frac{\text{Moments of gratitude expressed}}{\text{Total opportunities for gratitude}}$$

### 4.4.3 Connection with Nature Index

Strengthen spiritual connection with the Nature Bonding Quotient ($NBQ$):

$$NBQ = \frac{\text{Quality moments spent in nature}}{\text{Total time in natural surroundings}}$$

### 4.4.4 Compassion in Action

Express compassion with the Compassion Manifestation Score ($CMS$):

$$CMS = \frac{\text{Acts of kindness and compassion}}{\text{Total opportunities for compassionate actions}}$$

### 4.4.5 Mindful Silence Efficiency

Enhance spiritual resilience with the Silence Awareness Quotient ($SAQ$):

$$SAQ = \frac{\text{Moments of mindful silence}}{\text{Total moments without external distractions}}$$

### 4.4.6 Sacred Ritual Integration

Integrate sacred rituals with the Ritual Alignment Index ($RAI$):

$$RAI = \frac{\text{Meaningful rituals practiced}}{\text{Total ritual opportunities}}$$

### 4.4.7 Transcendental Meditation Impact

Experience transcendence with the Transcendental Meditation Effectiveness ($TME$):

$$TME = \frac{\text{Positive impact of transcendental meditation}}{\text{Total meditation sessions}}$$

Spiritual resilience involves cultivating inner harmony through mindful reflection, gratitude, connection with nature, and sacred practices.

## 4.5 Overcoming Fear and Anxiety

Empowering oneself to overcome fear and anxiety involves practical insights and quantifiable measures for a resilient and calm mind.

### 4.5.1 Fear Confrontation Index

Confront fear with the Fear Mastery Quotient ($FMQ$):

$$FMQ = \frac{\text{Successfully faced fears}}{\text{Total fear-inducing situations}}$$

### 4.5.2 Anxiety Reduction Ratio

Reduce anxiety with the Anxiety Alleviation Index ($AAI$):

$$AAI = \frac{\text{Decrease in anxiety levels}}{\text{Total anxiety-triggered instances}}$$

### 4.5.3   Mindful Breathing Relief

Calm anxiety with the Breath Relaxation Efficiency ($BRE$):

$$BRE = \frac{\text{Anxiety-relieving breaths}}{\text{Total breaths during anxious moments}}$$

### 4.5.4   Positive Affirmation Shield

Shield against fear with the Affirmation Resilience Factor ($ARF$):

$$ARF = \frac{\text{Positive affirmations during fearful situations}}{\text{Instances of negative self-talk}}$$

### 4.5.5   Cognitive Restructuring Effectiveness

Restructure thoughts with the Cognitive Transformation Quotient ($CTQ$):

$$CTQ = \frac{\text{Successful cognitive restructuring instances}}{\text{Total cognitive restructuring attempts}}$$

### 4.5.6   Mind-Body Relaxation Coefficient

Relax the mind and body with the Relaxation Synergy Score ($RSS$):

$$RSS = \frac{\text{Mind and body relaxation instances}}{\text{Total stress-inducing situations}}$$

### 4.5.7   Fear Exposure Therapy Impact

Leverage exposure therapy with the Fear Exposure Effectiveness ($FEE$):

$$FEE = \frac{\text{Positive impact of fear exposure}}{\text{Total exposure therapy sessions}}$$

Overcoming fear and anxiety involves practical strategies to face fears, alleviate anxiety, and foster a calm and resilient mind.

## 4.6   Art and Expression in Healing

Engaging in art and expression for healing involves practical insights and quantifiable measures for fostering creativity and well-being.

### 4.6.1   Creative Expression Quotient

Measure creative expression with the Creativity Impact Index ($CII$):

$$CII = \frac{\text{Positive impact of creative expression}}{\text{Total creative expression instances}}$$

### 4.6.2   Artistic Satisfaction Ratio

Enhance satisfaction with artistic endeavors using the Artistic Fulfillment Quotient ($AFQ$):

$$AFQ = \frac{\text{Satisfaction derived from artistic activities}}{\text{Total time spent on artistic pursuits}}$$

### 4.6.3   Emotional Release Efficiency

Release emotions through art with the Emotional Artistry Coefficient ($EAC$):

$$EAC = \frac{\text{Effective emotional release through art}}{\text{Total emotional release attempts}}$$

### 4.6.4   Mindful Art Presence

Cultivate mindfulness through art with the Artful Mindfulness Index ($AMI$):

$$AMI = \frac{\text{Moments fully present during artistic activities}}{\text{Total time engaged in art}}$$

### 4.6.5   Therapeutic Art Impact

Leverage art for therapy with the Art Therapy Effectiveness ($ATE$):

$$ATE = \frac{\text{Positive impact of art therapy}}{\text{Total art therapy sessions}}$$

### 4.6.6   Creative Flow Optimization

Optimize creative flow with the Flow State Attainment ($FSA$):

$$FSA = \frac{\text{Moments of flow experienced during artistic activities}}{\text{Total time spent in creative pursuits}}$$

### 4.6.7   Artistic Reflection Depth

Deepen reflection through art with the Artful Reflection Index ($ARI$):

$$ARI = \frac{\text{Depth of reflection achieved through artistic endeavors}}{\text{Total time spent in reflection}}$$

Art and expression in healing involve fostering creativity, satisfaction, and emotional release for a holistic well-being.

## 4.7 Joyful Moments Amidst Challenges

Embracing joy amidst challenges involves practical insights and quantifiable measures for cultivating positivity and resilience.

### 4.7.1 Joy Resilience Quotient

Foster joy resilience with the Joyful Resilience Index ($JRI$):

$$JRI = \frac{\text{Positive moments amidst challenges}}{\text{Total challenging situations}}$$

### 4.7.2 Gratitude Amplification

Amplify joy through gratitude with the Gratitude Expansion Ratio ($GER$):

$$GER = \frac{\text{Moments of gratitude expressed}}{\text{Total opportunities for gratitude}}$$

### 4.7.3 Laughter Therapy Impact

Leverage laughter for therapy with the Laughter Resilience Coefficient ($LRC$):

$$LRC = \frac{\text{Positive impact of laughter on mood}}{\text{Total laughter-inducing situations}}$$

### 4.7.4 Positive Affirmation Boost

Uplift positivity with the Affirmation Resilience Factor ($ARF$):

$$ARF = \frac{\text{Positive affirmations internalized}}{\text{Instances of negative self-talk}}$$

### 4.7.5 Mindful Joy Infusion

Infuse mindfulness into joyful moments with the Joyful Mindfulness Quotient ($JMQ$):

$$JMQ = \frac{\text{Mindful presence during moments of joy}}{\text{Total joyful moments}}$$

### 4.7.6  Social Connection Synergy

Foster joy through social connections with the Social Joy Engagement ($SJE$):

$$SJE = \frac{\text{Quality interactions fostering joy}}{\text{Total social interactions}}$$

### 4.7.7  Humor Resilience Formula

Build resilience through humor with the Humor Resilience Efficiency ($HRE$):

$$HRE = \frac{\text{Effective use of humor in challenging situations}}{\text{Total challenging moments}}$$

Joyful moments amidst challenges involve cultivating positivity, gratitude, laughter, and mindful presence for resilient well-being.

# Chapter 5

# Survivorship and Beyond

## 5.1 Life After Treatment

Navigating life after treatment involves practical insights and quantifiable measures for a vibrant and resilient post-treatment journey.

### 5.1.1 Recovery Momentum Index

Measure recovery momentum with the Recovery Velocity Score ($RVS$):

$$RVS = \frac{\text{Speed of physical and emotional recovery}}{\text{Total recovery time}}$$

### 5.1.2 Reintegration Success Quotient

Ensure successful reintegration with the Reintegration Efficiency ($RE$):

$$RE = \frac{\text{Smooth reintegration into daily life}}{\text{Total reintegration challenges}}$$

### 5.1.3 Post-Traumatic Growth Formula

Promote growth after trauma with the Growth Resilience Index ($GRI$):

$$GRI = \frac{\text{Positive growth experiences}}{\text{Total post-treatment challenges}}$$

### 5.1.4  Wellness Sustenance Ratio

Sustain wellness with the Wellness Continuity Quotient ($WCQ$):

$$WCQ = \frac{\text{Consistency in maintaining wellness practices}}{\text{Total days post-treatment}}$$

### 5.1.5  Future Hopefulness Quotient

Cultivate hope for the future with the Hopeful Outlook Score ($HOS$):

$$HOS = \frac{\text{Positive thoughts about the future}}{\text{Total moments of uncertainty}}$$

### 5.1.6  Joyful Milestones Celebration

Celebrate milestones with the Milestone Achievement Index ($MAI$):

$$MAI = \frac{\text{Joyful moments marking achievements}}{\text{Total milestones post-treatment}}$$

### 5.1.7  Community Connection Synergy

Foster connection with the Survivor Community Engagement ($SCE$):

$$SCE = \frac{\text{Positive interactions within the survivor community}}{\text{Total community engagements}}$$

Life after treatment involves maintaining wellness, celebrating achievements, and embracing a hopeful and resilient future.

## 5.2  Follow-Up Care

Navigating follow-up care involves practical insights and quantifiable measures for continued well-being.

### 5.2.1  Health Monitoring Index

Monitor health with the Health Surveillance Quotient ($HSQ$):

$$HSQ = \frac{\text{Effectiveness of health monitoring}}{\text{Total health check instances}}$$

### 5.2.2  Wellness Check Compliance

Comply with wellness checks using the Wellness Check Adherence ($WCA$):

$$WCA = \frac{\text{Adherence to recommended wellness checks}}{\text{Total recommended wellness checks}}$$

### 5.2.3  Mind-Body Check Integration

Integrate mind-body checks with the Holistic Check Fusion ($HCF$):

$$HCF = \frac{\text{Mind and body checks integrated into routine}}{\text{Total routine check instances}}$$

### 5.2.4  Preventive Action Initiative

Take preventive actions with the Preventive Action Index ($PAI$):

$$PAI = \frac{\text{Proactive measures taken to prevent health issues}}{\text{Total preventive actions}}$$

### 5.2.5  Treatment Recovery Assessment

Assess recovery post-treatment with the Recovery Evaluation Quotient ($REQ$):

$$REQ = \frac{\text{Degree of recovery achieved}}{\text{Total post-treatment assessments}}$$

### 5.2.6  Lifestyle Adjustment Rating

Adjust lifestyle for well-being with the Lifestyle Adaptation Score ($LAS$):

$$LAS = \frac{\text{Positive lifestyle adjustments made}}{\text{Total lifestyle adjustment opportunities}}$$

### 5.2.7  Health Empowerment Quotient

Empower health decisions with the Health Empowerment ($HE$):

$$HE = \frac{\text{Degree of empowerment in health choices}}{\text{Total health decisions}}$$

Follow-up care involves proactive health monitoring, adherence to wellness checks, and empowered decision-making for continued well-being.

## 5.3 Embracing the "New Normal"

Embracing the "New Normal" involves practical insights and quantifiable measures for adapting positively to life post-treatment.

### 5.3.1 Adaptability Resilience

Enhance adaptability with the Adaptation Quotient ($AQ$):

$$AQ = \frac{\text{Successful adaptations to new circumstances}}{\text{Total instances of adapting to change}}$$

### 5.3.2 Mindful Presence in Change

Cultivate mindfulness during changes with the Change Awareness Score ($CAS$):

$$CAS = \frac{\text{Moments fully present during changes}}{\text{Total moments of change}}$$

### 5.3.3 Social Reintegration Index

Reintegrate socially with the Social Reintegration Quotient ($SRQ$):

$$SRQ = \frac{\text{Successful social reintegration instances}}{\text{Total social reintegration opportunities}}$$

### 5.3.4 Resilience in Routine Adjustments

Build resilience in routine adjustments with the Routine Resilience Coefficient ($RRC$):

$$RRC = \frac{\text{Positive response to routine changes}}{\text{Total routine changes}}$$

### 5.3.5 Positive Perspective Boost

Boost positivity with the Positivity Amplification Factor ($PAF$):

$$PAF = \frac{\text{Moments of positive perspective towards the 'New Normal'}}{\text{Total instances of facing the 'New Normal'}}$$

### 5.3.6 Community Connection Synergy

Forge connections within the community with the Community Connection Index ($CCI$):

$$CCI = \frac{\text{Quality interactions within the community}}{\text{Total community interaction opportunities}}$$

### 5.3.7 Mind-Body Wellness Alignment

Align mind and body wellness with the Wellness Synchronization ($WS$):

$$WS = \frac{\text{Balanced mind and body wellness in the 'New Normal'}}{\text{Total moments in the 'New Normal'}}$$

Embracing the "New Normal" involves fostering adaptability, mindfulness, social reintegration, and positive perspectives for a fulfilling post-treatment life.

## 5.4 Support for Long-Term Wellness

Ensuring long-term wellness involves practical insights and quantifiable measures for sustained support and health maintenance.

### 5.4.1 Holistic Wellness Check

Conduct a holistic wellness check with the Comprehensive Wellness Assessment ($CWA$):

$$CWA = \frac{\text{Overall wellness score}}{\text{Total wellness categories assessed}}$$

### 5.4.2 Social Support Index

Leverage social support with the Social Support Quotient ($SSQ$):

$$SSQ = \frac{\text{Quality social interactions fostering support}}{\text{Total social interaction opportunities}}$$

### 5.4.3 Personal Wellness Plan

Craft a personalized wellness plan with the Personal Wellness Blueprint ($PWB$):

$$PWB = \frac{\text{Effectiveness of personal wellness plan implementation}}{\text{Total wellness plan adjustments}}$$

### 5.4.4 Mindful Self-Care Practices

Engage in mindful self-care with the Mindful Self-Care Efficiency ($MSCE$):

$$MSCE = \frac{\text{Effective moments of mindful self-care}}{\text{Total self-care instances}}$$

### 5.4.5 Nutrient-Rich Lifestyle

Maintain a nutrient-rich lifestyle with the Nutrient Integration Quotient ($NIQ$):

$$NIQ = \frac{\text{Nutrient-dense choices made}}{\text{Total daily lifestyle choices}}$$

### 5.4.6 Physical Activity Sustainability

Sustain physical activity with the Exercise Longevity Ratio ($ELR$):

$$ELR = \frac{\text{Consistency in physical activity over time}}{\text{Total days of physical activity}}$$

### 5.4.7 Mental Resilience Boost

Boost mental resilience with the Mental Resilience Index ($MRI$):

$$MRI = \frac{\text{Positive mental resilience instances}}{\text{Total challenging mental situations}}$$

Support for long-term wellness involves a holistic approach encompassing physical, social, and mental well-being for sustained health and happiness.

## 5.5 Relationships Post-Treatment

Navigating relationships post-treatment involves practical insights and quantifiable measures for fostering connections and understanding.

### 5.5.1 Communication Harmony Quotient

Cultivate communication harmony with the Communication Synchronization ($CS$):

$$CS = \frac{\text{Effective communication instances}}{\text{Total communication opportunities}}$$

### 5.5.2 Empathy Amplification Factor

Amplify empathy within relationships using the Empathy Boost ($EB$):

$$EB = \frac{\text{Moments of heightened empathy}}{\text{Total empathetic instances}}$$

### 5.5.3 Quality Time Integration

Integrate quality time into relationships with the Quality Time Fusion ($QTF$):

$$QTF = \frac{\text{Quality time spent together}}{\text{Total time spent in relationship activities}}$$

### 5.5.4 Conflict Resolution Efficiency

Resolve conflicts efficiently using the Conflict Resolution Effectiveness ($CRE$):

$$CRE = \frac{\text{Positive conflict resolution instances}}{\text{Total conflict situations}}$$

### 5.5.5 Affectionate Gestures Ratio

Express affection with the Affection Amplification ($AA$):

$$AA = \frac{\text{Affectionate gestures and expressions}}{\text{Total opportunities for affection}}$$

### 5.5.6 Shared Goals Alignment

Align on shared goals with the Goal Synchronization ($GS$):

$$GS = \frac{\text{Agreement on shared goals}}{\text{Total shared goals discussions}}$$

### 5.5.7 Relationship Growth Index

Measure relationship growth with the Relationship Expansion Quotient ($REQ$):

$$REQ = \frac{\text{Positive relationship growth instances}}{\text{Total relationship growth opportunities}}$$

Relationships post-treatment involve effective communication, empathy, quality time, conflict resolution, affection, shared goals, and continuous growth for a fulfilling connection.

## 5.6 Career and Financial Considerations

Navigating career and financial aspects post-treatment involves practical insights and quantifiable measures for stability and growth.

### 5.6.1   Financial Health Assessment

Assess financial health with the Financial Stability Index ($FSI$):

$$FSI = \frac{\text{Overall financial stability}}{\text{Total financial assessments}}$$

### 5.6.2   Career Satisfaction Quotient

Measure career satisfaction with the Career Fulfillment Ratio ($CFR$):

$$CFR = \frac{\text{Satisfaction derived from work}}{\text{Total work-related instances}}$$

### 5.6.3   Budgeting Efficiency

Optimize budgeting with the Budget Management Score ($BMS$):

$$BMS = \frac{\text{Effective budget management instances}}{\text{Total budgeting opportunities}}$$

### 5.6.4   Financial Growth Potential

Explore financial growth with the Financial Expansion Quotient ($FEQ$):

$$FEQ = \frac{\text{Potential for financial growth}}{\text{Total financial planning discussions}}$$

### 5.6.5   Career Development Impact

Leverage career development with the Career Advancement Efficiency ($CAE$):

$$CAE = \frac{\text{Positive impact on career development}}{\text{Total career development opportunities}}$$

### 5.6.6   Investment Wisdom Ratio

Apply investment wisdom with the Investment Strategy Effectiveness ($ISE$):

$$ISE = \frac{\text{Effectiveness of investment decisions}}{\text{Total investment opportunities}}$$

### 5.6.7   Emergency Fund Resilience

Build resilience with an emergency fund using the Emergency Preparedness Quotient ($EPQ$):

$$EPQ = \frac{\text{Emergency fund effectiveness}}{\text{Total emergency situations}}$$

Career and financial considerations post-treatment involve maintaining stability, finding fulfillment in work, effective budgeting, planning for growth, and making wise financial decisions.

## 5.7  Celebrating Milestones

Celebrating milestones post-treatment involves practical insights and quantifiable measures for acknowledging achievements and fostering positivity.

### 5.7.1  Milestone Achievement Rate

Acknowledge milestone achievements with the Milestone Success Rate ($MSR$):

$$MSR = \frac{\text{Successful milestone celebrations}}{\text{Total milestone opportunities}}$$

### 5.7.2  Gratitude Integration Quotient

Integrate gratitude into celebrations with the Gratitude Amplification ($GA$):

$$GA = \frac{\text{Moments of gratitude during celebrations}}{\text{Total celebratory occasions}}$$

### 5.7.3  Positive Reflection Boost

Boost positivity with the Reflection Positivity Factor ($RPF$):

$$RPF = \frac{\text{Positive reflection during milestones}}{\text{Total milestone reflections}}$$

### 5.7.4  Self-Appreciation Rating

Encourage self-appreciation with the Self-Recognition Index ($SRI$):

$$SRI = \frac{\text{Instances of self-appreciation}}{\text{Total opportunities for self-recognition}}$$

### 5.7.5  Community Appreciation Index

Feel appreciated within the community with the Community Recognition Quotient ($CRQ$):

$$CRQ = \frac{\text{Positive community recognition}}{\text{Total community interaction opportunities}}$$

### 5.7.6  Joyful Achievement Amplification

Amplify joy in achievements with the Achievement Joy Multiplier ($AJM$):

$$AJM = \frac{\text{Moments of joy during milestone achievements}}{\text{Total achievements celebrated}}$$

### 5.7.7  Life Satisfaction Elevation

Elevate life satisfaction with the Satisfaction Ascendancy ($SA$):

$$SA = \frac{\text{Positive life satisfaction instances}}{\text{Total moments of life satisfaction}}$$

Celebrating milestones involves acknowledging achievements, fostering gratitude, positive reflection, self-appreciation, community recognition, joyful amplification, and elevating overall life satisfaction.

# Chapter 6

# Empowering Others

## 6.1 Becoming an Advocate

Becoming an advocate involves practical insights and quantifiable measures for making a positive impact and empowering others.

### 6.1.1 Advocacy Impact Score

Measure advocacy impact with the Advocacy Effectiveness ($AE$):

$$AE = \frac{\text{Positive impact of advocacy efforts}}{\text{Total advocacy initiatives}}$$

### 6.1.2 Communication Influence Quotient

Influence through communication with the Communication Advocacy Index ($CAI$):

$$CAI = \frac{\text{Effective communication in advocacy}}{\text{Total communication instances in advocacy}}$$

### 6.1.3 Policy Change Efficiency

Drive policy change efficiently with the Policy Advocacy Efficiency ($PAE$):

$$PAE = \frac{\text{Effectiveness in driving policy change}}{\text{Total policy change initiatives}}$$

### 6.1.4 Community Engagement Rating

Engage the community with the Community Advocacy Engagement ($CAE$):

$$CAE = \frac{\text{Quality community interactions in advocacy}}{\text{Total community engagement opportunities}}$$

### 6.1.5 Educational Impact Quotient

Measure educational impact with the Advocacy Education Quotient ($AEQ$):

$$AEQ = \frac{\text{Positive educational impact through advocacy}}{\text{Total educational initiatives in advocacy}}$$

### 6.1.6 Positive Change Multiplier

Multiply positive change with the Advocacy Change Amplification ($ACA$):

$$ACA = \frac{\text{Amplification of positive change through advocacy}}{\text{Total instances of positive change}}$$

### 6.1.7 Empowerment Uplift

Uplift empowerment with the Advocacy Empowerment Factor ($AEF$):

$$AEF = \frac{\text{Empowerment impact of advocacy}}{\text{Total instances of empowerment}}$$

Becoming an advocate involves making a positive impact through effective communication, driving policy change, engaging the community, educational initiatives, amplifying positive change, and uplifting empowerment.

## 6.2 Supporting Loved Ones

Supporting loved ones involves practical insights and quantifiable measures for providing meaningful assistance and fostering well-being.

### 6.2.1 Caregiver Resilience Index

Measure caregiver resilience with the Caregiver Resilience Quotient ($CRQ$):

$$CRQ = \frac{\text{Resilience demonstrated by the caregiver}}{\text{Total caregiving situations}}$$

### 6.2.2 Empathy Amplification Factor

Amplify empathy in support with the Empathy Boost ($EB$):

$$EB = \frac{\text{Moments of heightened empathy during support}}{\text{Total instances of providing support}}$$

### 6.2.3 Quality Time Integration

Integrate quality time into support with the Quality Time Fusion ($QTF$):

$$QTF = \frac{\text{Quality time spent with loved ones}}{\text{Total time spent in supporting activities}}$$

### 6.2.4 Positive Reflection Boost

Boost positivity with the Reflection Positivity Factor ($RPF$):

$$RPF = \frac{\text{Positive reflection during support moments}}{\text{Total moments of providing support}}$$

### 6.2.5 Affectionate Gestures Ratio

Express affection in support with the Affection Amplification ($AA$):

$$AA = \frac{\text{Affectionate gestures and expressions during support}}{\text{Total opportunities for providing support}}$$

### 6.2.6 Shared Goals Alignment

Align on shared goals with loved ones through the Goal Synchronization ($GS$):

$$GS = \frac{\text{Agreement on shared goals during support}}{\text{Total shared goals discussions in support}}$$

### 6.2.7 Well-Being Uplift

Uplift well-being with the Supportive Well-Being Factor ($SWBF$):

$$SWBF = \frac{\text{Positive impact on well-being through support}}{\text{Total instances of providing support}}$$

Supporting loved ones involves demonstrating resilience, empathy, quality time, positive reflection, affection, shared goals, and uplifting overall well-being.

## 6.3   Community Outreach

Engaging in community outreach involves practical insights and quantifiable measures for making a positive impact and fostering collective well-being.

### 6.3.1   Community Impact Score

Measure impact on the community with the Community Well-Being Index ($CWI$):

$$CWI = \frac{\text{Positive impact on community well-being}}{\text{Total community outreach initiatives}}$$

### 6.3.2   Connection Amplification Factor

Amplify connections within the community with the Connection Boost ($CB$):

$$CB = \frac{\text{Moments of enhanced community connections}}{\text{Total community interactions}}$$

### 6.3.3   Quality Collaboration Ratio

Collaborate effectively with the Quality Collaboration Index ($QCI$):

$$QCI = \frac{\text{Effective collaboration in community initiatives}}{\text{Total collaborative opportunities}}$$

### 6.3.4   Positive Change Multiplier

Multiply positive change with the Community Change Amplification ($CCA$):

$$CCA = \frac{\text{Amplification of positive change in the community}}{\text{Total instances of positive change}}$$

### 6.3.5   Educational Impact Quotient

Measure educational impact with the Community Education Quotient ($CEQ$):

$$CEQ = \frac{\text{Positive educational impact in the community}}{\text{Total educational initiatives in the community}}$$

### 6.3.6   Resource Utilization Efficiency

Utilize resources efficiently with the Resource Efficiency Quotient ($REQ$):

$$REQ = \frac{\text{Efficiency in resource utilization for community initiatives}}{\text{Total resources used}}$$

### 6.3.7 Empowerment Uplift

Uplift empowerment in the community with the Community Empowerment Factor ($CEF$):

$$CEF = \frac{\text{Empowerment impact on the community}}{\text{Total instances of community empowerment}}$$

Community outreach involves making a positive impact on well-being, amplifying connections, effective collaboration, multiplying positive change, educational impact, efficient resource utilization, and uplifting community empowerment.

## 6.4 Education Initiatives

Taking on education initiatives involves practical insights and quantifiable measures for fostering learning and empowering others.

### 6.4.1 Educational Impact Score

Measure impact on education with the Educational Empowerment Index ($EEI$):

$$EEI = \frac{\text{Positive impact on education initiatives}}{\text{Total education empowerment opportunities}}$$

### 6.4.2 Knowledge Amplification Factor

Amplify knowledge with the Knowledge Boost ($KB$):

$$KB = \frac{\text{Moments of heightened knowledge transfer}}{\text{Total educational interactions}}$$

### 6.4.3 Skill Development Quotient

Develop skills effectively with the Skill Enhancement Ratio ($SER$):

$$SER = \frac{\text{Effective skill development instances}}{\text{Total skill development opportunities}}$$

### 6.4.4 Positive Learning Multiplier

Multiply positive learning experiences with the Learning Amplification ($LA$):

$$LA = \frac{\text{Amplification of positive learning outcomes}}{\text{Total instances of positive learning}}$$

### 6.4.5　Innovation Integration Index

Integrate innovation in education with the Innovation Adoption ($IA$):

$$IA = \frac{\text{Effective adoption of innovative teaching methods}}{\text{Total opportunities for innovation in education}}$$

### 6.4.6　Resource Utilization Efficiency

Utilize educational resources efficiently with the Educational Resource Quotient ($ERQ$):

$$ERQ = \frac{\text{Efficiency in resource utilization for education}}{\text{Total resources used in education initiatives}}$$

### 6.4.7　Empowerment Uplift

Uplift empowerment through education with the Educational Empowerment Factor ($EEF$):

$$EEF = \frac{\text{Empowerment impact through education initiatives}}{\text{Total instances of empowerment in education}}$$

Education initiatives involve making a positive impact, amplifying knowledge, effective skill development, multiplying positive learning experiences, innovation integration, efficient resource utilization, and uplifting empowerment through education.

## 6.5　Volunteer Opportunities

Engaging in volunteer opportunities involves practical insights and quantifiable measures for making a positive impact and contributing to the community.

### 6.5.1　Impactful Contribution Index

Measure impact with the Contribution Effectiveness ($CE$):

$$CE = \frac{\text{Impactful contributions made}}{\text{Total volunteer opportunities}}$$

### 6.5.2　Time Utilization Efficiency

Utilize time efficiently with the Time Efficiency Quotient ($TEQ$):

$$TEQ = \frac{\text{Efficient use of time in volunteering}}{\text{Total time spent in volunteer activities}}$$

### 6.5.3 Skill Enhancement Quotient

Enhance skills through volunteering with the Skill Development Ratio ($SDR$):

$$SDR = \frac{\text{Effective skill development instances in volunteering}}{\text{Total skill enhancement opportunities}}$$

### 6.5.4 Positive Engagement Multiplier

Multiply positive engagement with the Engagement Amplification ($EA$):

$$EA = \frac{\text{Amplification of positive engagement in volunteer activities}}{\text{Total instances of positive engagement}}$$

### 6.5.5 Community Impact Integration

Integrate community impact with the Community Empowerment ($CEM$):

$$CEM = \frac{\text{Effective integration of community impact}}{\text{Total community empowerment initiatives}}$$

### 6.5.6 Resource Utilization Efficiency

Utilize resources efficiently with the Resource Efficiency ($RE$):

$$RE = \frac{\text{Efficiency in resource utilization for volunteering}}{\text{Total resources used in volunteer activities}}$$

### 6.5.7 Empowerment Uplift

Uplift empowerment through volunteering with the Volunteering Empowerment ($VE$):

$$VE = \frac{\text{Empowerment impact through volunteering}}{\text{Total instances of empowerment in volunteering}}$$

Volunteer opportunities involve making impactful contributions, efficient time utilization, skill enhancement, multiplying positive engagement, integrating community impact, resource utilization efficiency, and uplifting empowerment through volunteering.

## 6.6 Fostering Hope in Others

Fostering hope in others involves practical insights and quantifiable measures for uplifting spirits and instilling positivity.

### 6.6.1 Hope Amplification Index

Amplify hope with the Hope Boost ($HB$):

$$HB = \frac{\text{Moments of heightened hope in others}}{\text{Total instances of fostering hope}}$$

### 6.6.2 Positivity Uplift Quotient

Uplift positivity with the Positivity Ascendancy ($PA$):

$$PA = \frac{\text{Positive impact on others' outlook}}{\text{Total opportunities for fostering hope}}$$

### 6.6.3 Resilience Reinforcement Ratio

Reinforce resilience with the Resilience Enhancement ($RE$):

$$RE = \frac{\text{Effective reinforcement of resilience in others}}{\text{Total instances of resilience building}}$$

### 6.6.4 Joyful Moments Integration

Integrate joyful moments with the Joy Amplification ($JA$):

$$JA = \frac{\text{Amplification of joy in others}}{\text{Total instances of fostering joy}}$$

### 6.6.5 Encouragement Multiplier

Multiply encouragement with the Encouragement Amplification ($EA$):

$$EA = \frac{\text{Amplification of encouragement in others}}{\text{Total instances of providing encouragement}}$$

### 6.6.6 Positive Affirmation Efficiency

Affirm positivity efficiently with the Affirmation Quotient ($AQ$):

$$AQ = \frac{\text{Efficiency in affirming positive outcomes}}{\text{Total positive affirmations shared}}$$

### 6.6.7 Empowerment Uplift

Uplift empowerment through fostering hope with the Hopeful Empowerment ($HE$):

$$HE = \frac{\text{Empowerment impact through fostering hope}}{\text{Total instances of empowerment through hope}}$$

Fostering hope in others involves amplifying hope, uplifting positivity, reinforcing resilience, integrating joyful moments, multiplying encouragement, efficient positive affirmation, and uplifting empowerment through hope.

## 6.7 Continuing the Fight Against Cancer

Continuing the fight against cancer involves practical insights and quantifiable measures for sustained efforts and positive impact.

### 6.7.1 Impactful Advocacy Index

Measure impact in advocacy with the Advocacy Impact ($AI$):

$$AI = \frac{\text{Sustained impactful advocacy efforts}}{\text{Total advocacy initiatives over time}}$$

### 6.7.2 Community Resilience Ratio

Build community resilience with the Resilience Building ($RB$):

$$RB = \frac{\text{Effective community resilience initiatives}}{\text{Total resilience-building programs}}$$

### 6.7.3 Educational Continuity Quotient

Ensure educational continuity with the Education Continuity ($EC$):

$$EC = \frac{\text{Continuous positive impact on cancer education}}{\text{Total educational initiatives over time}}$$

### 6.7.4 Hopefulness Sustainment Factor

Sustain hopefulness with the Hopefulness Sustainment ($HS$):

$$HS = \frac{\text{Consistent positive impact on fostering hope}}{\text{Total instances of fostering hope over time}}$$

### 6.7.5 Volunteerism Persistence Ratio

Persist in volunteer efforts with the Volunteerism Persistence ($VP$):

$$VP = \frac{\text{Persistent impactful volunteer opportunities}}{\text{Total volunteer opportunities over time}}$$

### 6.7.6  Innovation Integration Index

Integrate innovation in the fight with the Innovation Integration ($II$):

$$II = \frac{\text{Continuous adoption of innovative approaches}}{\text{Total instances of innovation in the fight}}$$

### 6.7.7  Empowerment Continuity

Ensure empowerment continuity with the Empowerment Continuity ($EC$):

$$EC = \frac{\text{Continuous positive impact on empowerment}}{\text{Total instances of empowerment over time}}$$

Continuing the fight against cancer involves sustained impactful advocacy, building community resilience, ensuring educational continuity, sustaining hopefulness, persisting in volunteer efforts, continuous innovation, and ensuring empowerment continuity.

# Chapter 7

# Facing Recurrence

## 7.1 Understanding Recurrence

Facing recurrence involves a practical understanding to navigate challenges and make informed decisions.

### 7.1.1 Recurrence Risk Assessment

Assess the risk of recurrence with the Recurrence Probability ($RP$):

$$RP = \frac{\text{Number of recurrences}}{\text{Total cases studied}}$$

### 7.1.2 Tumor Progression Rate

Evaluate tumor progression rate with the Progression Index ($PI$):

$$PI = \frac{\text{Rate of tumor growth}}{\text{Time elapsed since initial treatment}}$$

### 7.1.3 Early Detection Importance

Understand the importance of early detection with the Early Identification Quotient ($EIQ$):

$$EIQ = \frac{\text{Effectiveness in early identification}}{\text{Total instances of recurrence}}$$

### 7.1.4  Treatment Response Analysis

Analyze treatment responses with the Response Evaluation ($RE$):

$$RE = \frac{\text{Positive treatment responses}}{\text{Total recurrence treatment instances}}$$

### 7.1.5  Genetic and Environmental Factors

Consider genetic and environmental factors in recurrence with the Risk Influencing Factors ($RIF$):

$$RIF = \frac{\text{Genetic and environmental factors contributing to recurrence}}{\text{Total factors studied}}$$

### 7.1.6  Psychosocial Impact

Assess psychosocial impact with the Psychosocial Burden Score ($PBS$):

$$PBS = \frac{\text{Psychosocial burden experienced}}{\text{Total instances of recurrence impact}}$$

### 7.1.7  Empowerment Through Knowledge

Empower through knowledge with the Knowledge Empowerment ($KE$):

$$KE = \frac{\text{Empowerment impact through understanding recurrence}}{\text{Total instances of knowledge empowerment}}$$

Understanding recurrence involves assessing risks, evaluating progression, emphasizing early detection, analyzing treatment responses, considering influencing factors, assessing psychosocial impact, and empowering through knowledge.

## 7.2  Emotional Impact of Recurrence

Facing the emotional impact of recurrence involves understanding and managing the psychological challenges that may arise.

### 7.2.1  Emotional Resilience Quotient

Strengthen emotional resilience with the Resilience Index ($RI$):

$$RI = \frac{\text{Moments of emotional resilience}}{\text{Total emotional challenges faced}}$$

### 7.2.2  Anxiety Reduction Techniques

Implement anxiety reduction techniques with the Anxiety Alleviation Score ($AAS$):

$$AAS = \frac{\text{Effectiveness in reducing anxiety}}{\text{Total instances of anxiety management}}$$

### 7.2.3  Depression Mitigation Strategies

Utilize depression mitigation strategies with the Depression Relief Index ($DRI$):

$$DRI = \frac{\text{Effectiveness in mitigating depression}}{\text{Total instances of depression management}}$$

### 7.2.4  Coping Mechanism Efficiency

Evaluate coping mechanisms with the Coping Effectiveness Quotient ($CEQ$):

$$CEQ = \frac{\text{Efficiency in coping with emotional challenges}}{\text{Total instances of employing coping mechanisms}}$$

### 7.2.5  Support System Integration

Integrate support systems effectively with the Support Utilization Ratio ($SUR$):

$$SUR = \frac{\text{Effectiveness in utilizing emotional support}}{\text{Total opportunities for support utilization}}$$

### 7.2.6  Mindfulness and Well-being

Enhance mindfulness for improved well-being with the Mindful Living Score ($MLS$):

$$MLS = \frac{\text{Effectiveness in practicing mindfulness}}{\text{Total instances of mindfulness practice}}$$

### 7.2.7  Empowerment Through Emotional Understanding

Empower through emotional understanding with the Emotional Empowerment ($EE$):

$$EE = \frac{\text{Empowerment impact through understanding emotional challenges}}{\text{Total instances of emotional understanding empowerment}}$$

Facing the emotional impact of recurrence involves building resilience, alleviating anxiety, mitigating depression, efficient coping, effective support integration, practicing mindfulness, and empowering through emotional understanding.

## 7.3   Treatment Options for Recurrence

Exploring treatment options for recurrence involves practical considerations and understanding available interventions.

### 7.3.1   Treatment Efficacy Score

Assess treatment efficacy with the Efficacy Index ($EI$):

$$EI = \frac{\text{Positive treatment outcomes}}{\text{Total instances of treatment for recurrence}}$$

### 7.3.2   Survival Rate Improvement

Improve survival rates with the Survival Enhancement Quotient ($SEQ$):

$$SEQ = \frac{\text{Improvement in survival rates}}{\text{Total instances of recurrence survival improvement}}$$

### 7.3.3   Side Effect Management

Effectively manage side effects with the Side Effect Mitigation Score ($SMS$):

$$SMS = \frac{\text{Effectiveness in mitigating treatment side effects}}{\text{Total instances of side effect management}}$$

### 7.3.4   Treatment Personalization

Personalize treatments with the Personalization Quotient ($PQ$):

$$PQ = \frac{\text{Effectiveness in personalized treatment approaches}}{\text{Total instances of personalized treatment}}$$

### 7.3.5   Innovative Therapies Integration

Integrate innovative therapies with the Innovation Utilization Index ($IUI$):

$$IUI = \frac{\text{Effective integration of innovative therapies}}{\text{Total opportunities for innovative treatments}}$$

### 7.3.6   Quality of Life Enhancement

Enhance quality of life during treatment with the Quality Living Score ($QLS$):

$$QLS = \frac{\text{Improvement in quality of life during treatment}}{\text{Total instances of quality of life enhancement}}$$

### 7.3.7 Empowerment Through Informed Decisions

Empower through informed decisions with the Informed Empowerment ($IE$):

$$IE = \frac{\text{Empowerment impact through understanding treatment options}}{\text{Total instances of informed decision-making}}$$

Exploring treatment options for recurrence involves assessing efficacy, improving survival rates, managing side effects, personalizing treatments, integrating innovative therapies, enhancing quality of life, and empowering through informed decisions.

## 7.4 Coping Strategies for Ongoing Challenges

Navigating ongoing challenges during recurrence involves practical coping strategies and resilience-building.

### 7.4.1 Resilience Reinforcement Quotient

Strengthen resilience with the Resilience Boost ($RB$):

$$RB = \frac{\text{Instances of resilience reinforcement}}{\text{Total ongoing challenges faced}}$$

### 7.4.2 Stress Reduction Techniques

Implement stress reduction techniques with the Stress Alleviation Score ($SAS$):

$$SAS = \frac{\text{Effectiveness in reducing stress}}{\text{Total instances of stress management}}$$

### 7.4.3 Adaptability Enhancement

Enhance adaptability with the Adaptability Quotient ($AQ$):

$$AQ = \frac{\text{Improvement in adaptability to ongoing challenges}}{\text{Total adaptability enhancement opportunities}}$$

### 7.4.4 Mindfulness Practices Integration

Integrate mindfulness practices with the Mindful Coping Index ($MCI$):

$$MCI = \frac{\text{Effective integration of mindfulness practices}}{\text{Total instances of mindful coping}}$$

### 7.4.5  Social Support Utilization

Utilize social support effectively with the Social Support Quotient ($SSQ$):

$$SSQ = \frac{\text{Effectiveness in utilizing social support networks}}{\text{Total instances of social support utilization}}$$

### 7.4.6  Positive Affirmation Implementation

Implement positive affirmations with the Affirmation Integration ($AI$):

$$AI = \frac{\text{Integration of positive affirmations in daily life}}{\text{Total instances of positive affirmation usage}}$$

### 7.4.7  Empowerment Through Resilience

Empower through resilience with the Resilience Empowerment ($RE$):

$$RE = \frac{\text{Empowerment impact through resilience-building}}{\text{Total instances of empowerment through resilience}}$$

Navigating ongoing challenges during recurrence involves strengthening resilience, implementing stress reduction techniques, enhancing adaptability, integrating mindfulness practices, utilizing social support, implementing positive affirmations, and empowering through resilience.

## 7.5  Building a Renewed Support System

Building a renewed support system during recurrence involves practical strategies to strengthen your network.

### 7.5.1  Support Network Expansion

Expand your support network with the Network Growth Index ($NGI$):

$$NGI = \frac{\text{Growth in support network size}}{\text{Total instances of network expansion}}$$

### 7.5.2  Effective Communication Strategies

Implement effective communication with the Communication Mastery Score ($CMS$):

$$CMS = \frac{\text{Effectiveness in communication within the support system}}{\text{Total instances of effective communication}}$$

### 7.5.3   Understanding Emotional Needs

Meet emotional needs with the Emotional Understanding Ratio ($EUR$):

$$EUR = \frac{\text{Understanding emotional needs within the support system}}{\text{Total instances of emotional support}}$$

### 7.5.4   Shared Decision-Making

Engage in shared decision-making with the Decision Collaboration Quotient ($DCQ$):

$$DCQ = \frac{\text{Collaboration in decision-making within the support system}}{\text{Total instances of shared decision-making}}$$

### 7.5.5   Practical Assistance Utilization

Utilize practical assistance effectively with the Assistance Utilization Score ($AUS$):

$$AUS = \frac{\text{Effectiveness in utilizing practical support}}{\text{Total instances of practical assistance}}$$

### 7.5.6   Positive Environment Cultivation

Cultivate a positive environment with the Positivity Cultivation Index ($PCI$):

$$PCI = \frac{\text{Effectiveness in cultivating positivity within the support system}}{\text{Total instances of positivity cultivation}}$$

### 7.5.7   Empowerment Through Support

Empower through support with the Support Empowerment ($SE$):

$$SE = \frac{\text{Empowerment impact through building a renewed support system}}{\text{Total instances of empowerment through support}}$$

Building a renewed support system during recurrence involves expanding your network, mastering communication, understanding emotional needs, engaging in shared decision-making, utilizing practical assistance, cultivating a positive environment, and empowering through support.

## 7.6   Hope in the Face of Uncertainty

Finding hope amidst uncertainty involves practical approaches to maintain optimism and resilience.

### 7.6.1 Hope Resilience Index

Strengthen hope resilience with the Hope Resilience Quotient ($HRQ$):

$$HRQ = \frac{\text{Resilience in maintaining hope amidst uncertainty}}{\text{Total instances of facing uncertainty}}$$

### 7.6.2 Mindset Transformation Techniques

Transform mindset with the Mindset Shift Score ($MSS$):

$$MSS = \frac{\text{Effectiveness in shifting mindset towards hope}}{\text{Total instances of mindset transformation}}$$

### 7.6.3 Goal Setting for Renewed Focus

Set goals for renewed focus with the Goal Clarity Index ($GCI$):

$$GCI = \frac{\text{Clarity in setting and pursuing goals}}{\text{Total instances of goal setting}}$$

### 7.6.4 Cultivating Positivity

Cultivate positivity with the Positivity Amplification ($PA$):

$$PA = \frac{\text{Amplification of positivity amidst uncertainty}}{\text{Total instances of cultivating positivity}}$$

### 7.6.5 Self-Reflection for Resilience

Enhance resilience through self-reflection with the Resilient Self-Reflection ($RSR$):

$$RSR = \frac{\text{Impact of self-reflection on resilience}}{\text{Total instances of self-reflection}}$$

### 7.6.6 Connecting with Inspirational Figures

Connect with inspiration through figures with the Inspiration Link ($IL$):

$$IL = \frac{\text{Impact of connecting with inspirational figures}}{\text{Total instances of connection with inspiration}}$$

### 7.6.7 Empowerment Through Hope

Empower through hope with the Hope Empowerment ($HE$):

$$HE = \frac{\text{Empowerment impact through maintaining hope}}{\text{Total instances of empowerment through hope}}$$

Finding hope in the face of uncertainty involves strengthening hope resilience, transforming mindset, setting goals, cultivating positivity, self-reflection, connecting with inspiration, and empowering through hope.

## 7.7 Navigating Palliative Care

Navigating palliative care during recurrence involves practical considerations and understanding available support.

### 7.7.1 Palliative Care Utilization Index

Utilize palliative care effectively with the Palliative Care Index ($PCI$):

$$PCI = \frac{\text{Effectiveness in utilizing palliative care services}}{\text{Total instances of palliative care utilization}}$$

### 7.7.2 Quality of Life Enhancement

Enhance quality of life through palliative care with the Quality Living Score ($QLS$):

$$QLS = \frac{\text{Improvement in quality of life through palliative care}}{\text{Total instances of quality of life enhancement}}$$

### 7.7.3 Symptom Management Efficiency

Manage symptoms efficiently with the Symptom Relief Quotient ($SRQ$):

$$SRQ = \frac{\text{Efficiency in relieving symptoms through palliative care}}{\text{Total instances of symptom management}}$$

### 7.7.4 Emotional Support Integration

Integrate emotional support in palliative care with the Emotional Palliation Score ($EPS$):

$$EPS = \frac{\text{Effectiveness in emotional support during palliative care}}{\text{Total instances of emotional support integration}}$$

### 7.7.5 Collaborative Decision-Making

Engage in collaborative decision-making with the Collaborative Care Quotient ($CCQ$):

$$CCQ = \frac{\text{Collaboration in decision-making for palliative care}}{\text{Total instances of collaborative decision-making}}$$

### 7.7.6  Patient and Caregiver Education

Educate patients and caregivers with the Knowledge Empowerment ($KE$):

$$KE = \frac{\text{Empowerment through knowledge in palliative care}}{\text{Total instances of education in palliative care}}$$

### 7.7.7  Empowerment Through Palliative Care

Empower through palliative care with the Palliative Empowerment ($PE$):

$$PE = \frac{\text{Empowerment impact through navigating palliative care}}{\text{Total instances of empowerment through palliative care}}$$

Navigating palliative care during recurrence involves effective utilization, quality of life enhancement, symptom management, emotional support, collaborative decision-making, patient and caregiver education, and empowerment through palliative care.

# Chapter 8

# Inspiring Stories of Triumph

## 8.1 Profiles in Resilience

Explore real and practical stories of resilience through mathematical formulas capturing key aspects.

### 8.1.1 Resilience Index

Measure resilience with the Resilience Index ($RI$):

$$RI = \frac{\text{Overall resilience displayed in the story}}{\text{Total instances of resilience in the profile}}$$

### 8.1.2 Challenges Overcome Ratio

Quantify challenges overcome with the Challenges Conquered Quotient ($CCQ$):

$$CCQ = \frac{\text{Challenges conquered in the story}}{\text{Total instances of challenges faced}}$$

### 8.1.3 Growth and Transformation

Assess growth with the Growth and Transformation Score ($GTS$):

$$GTS = \frac{\text{Level of personal growth and transformation}}{\text{Total instances of growth and transformation}}$$

### 8.1.4 Support Network Impact

Evaluate support network impact with the Support Influence Index ($SII$):

$$SII = \frac{\text{Influence of support network on resilience}}{\text{Total instances of support network impact}}$$

### 8.1.5 Inspiration Quotient

Quantify inspiration with the Inspiration Quotient ($IQ$):

$$IQ = \frac{\text{Overall inspiration conveyed by the story}}{\text{Total instances of inspiration in the profile}}$$

### 8.1.6 Decision-Making Resilience

Assess decision-making resilience with the Decision Resilience ($DR$):

$$DR = \frac{\text{Resilience demonstrated in decision-making}}{\text{Total instances of decision-making resilience}}$$

### 8.1.7 Empowerment Through Adversity

Measure empowerment with the Adversity Empowerment ($AE$):

$$AE = \frac{\text{Empowerment impact through adversity}}{\text{Total instances of empowerment in the story}}$$

Explore profiles in resilience through the Resilience Index, Challenges Conquered Quotient, Growth and Transformation Score, Support Influence Index, Inspiration Quotient, Decision Resilience, and Adversity Empowerment.

## 8.2 Personal Journeys of Overcoming

Embark on inspiring journeys of overcoming challenges with practical metrics capturing key elements.

### 8.2.1 Overcoming Index

Quantify the ability to overcome challenges with the Overcoming Index ($OI$):

$$OI = \frac{\text{Overall success in overcoming challenges}}{\text{Total instances of challenges faced}}$$

### 8.2.2 Persistence Quotient

Measure persistence with the Persistence Quotient ($PQ$):

$$PQ = \frac{\text{Consistency in pursuing goals}}{\text{Total instances of persistence}}$$

### 8.2.3 Adaptability Resilience

Assess adaptability with the Adaptability Resilience ($AR$):

$$AR = \frac{\text{Resilience demonstrated in adapting to changing circumstances}}{\text{Total instances of adaptability}}$$

### 8.2.4 Learning Agility Impact

Evaluate learning agility with the Learning Agility Impact ($LAI$):

$$LAI = \frac{\text{Impact of learning from experiences}}{\text{Total instances of learning agility}}$$

### 8.2.5 Inspiration Coefficient

Quantify inspiration with the Inspiration Coefficient ($IC$):

$$IC = \frac{\text{Overall inspiration conveyed by the personal journey}}{\text{Total instances of inspiration in the story}}$$

### 8.2.6 Decision Resilience

Assess decision-making resilience with the Decision Resilience ($DR$):

$$DR = \frac{\text{Resilience demonstrated in decision-making}}{\text{Total instances of decision-making resilience}}$$

### 8.2.7 Empowerment Through Triumph

Measure empowerment with the Triumph Empowerment ($TE$):

$$TE = \frac{\text{Empowerment impact through personal triumph}}{\text{Total instances of empowerment in the story}}$$

Embark on personal journeys of overcoming with the Overcoming Index, Persistence Quotient, Adaptability Resilience, Learning Agility Impact, Inspiration Coefficient, Decision Resilience, and Triumph Empowerment.

## 8.3 Lessons from Survivors

Discover valuable lessons from survivors' experiences through practical metrics capturing key insights.

### 8.3.1 Resilience Impact Score

Quantify the impact of resilience with the Resilience Impact Score ($RIS$):

$$RIS = \frac{\text{Impact of resilience on overcoming challenges}}{\text{Total instances of resilience displayed}}$$

### 8.3.2 Wisdom Quotient

Measure wisdom with the Wisdom Quotient ($WQ$):

$$WQ = \frac{\text{Wisdom conveyed through lessons learned}}{\text{Total instances of wisdom in the story}}$$

### 8.3.3 Adversity Mastery Index

Assess mastery over adversity with the Adversity Mastery Index ($AMI$):

$$AMI = \frac{\text{Mastery demonstrated in facing and overcoming adversity}}{\text{Total instances of adversity mastery}}$$

### 8.3.4 Transformational Learning

Evaluate transformational learning with the Transformational Learning ($TL$):

$$TL = \frac{\text{Impact of learning experiences on personal transformation}}{\text{Total instances of transformational learning}}$$

### 8.3.5 Inspiration Catalyst

Quantify inspiration with the Inspiration Catalyst ($IC$):

$$IC = \frac{\text{Catalytic impact of lessons on inspiring others}}{\text{Total instances of inspiration in the story}}$$

### 8.3.6 Decision Wisdom

Assess decision-making wisdom with the Decision Wisdom ($DW$):

$$DW = \frac{\text{Wisdom displayed in decision-making}}{\text{Total instances of decision-making wisdom}}$$

### 8.3.7 Empowerment Through Lessons

Measure empowerment with the Lessons Empowerment ($LE$):

$$LE = \frac{\text{Empowerment impact through lessons learned}}{\text{Total instances of empowerment in the story}}$$

Discover lessons from survivors through the Resilience Impact Score, Wisdom Quotient, Adversity Mastery Index, Transformational Learning, Inspiration Catalyst, Decision Wisdom, and Lessons Empowerment.

## 8.4 Celebrating Courage

Celebrate extraordinary courage through real and practical metrics capturing the essence of inspiring stories.

### 8.4.1 Courage Quotient

Quantify courage with the Courage Quotient ($CQ$):

$$CQ = \frac{\text{Overall courage displayed in the story}}{\text{Total instances of courage exhibited}}$$

### 8.4.2 Fear Confrontation Index

Measure fear confrontation with the Fear Confrontation Index ($FCI$):

$$FCI = \frac{\text{Effectiveness in confronting and overcoming fear}}{\text{Total instances of fear confrontation}}$$

### 8.4.3 Bold Action Score

Assess bold actions with the Bold Action Score ($BAS$):

$$BAS = \frac{\text{Impact of bold actions on overcoming challenges}}{\text{Total instances of bold actions}}$$

### 8.4.4 Inspiration Cascade

Quantify inspiration with the Inspiration Cascade ($IC$):

$$IC = \frac{\text{Cascade effect of courage on inspiring others}}{\text{Total instances of inspiration in the story}}$$

### 8.4.5　Adversity Conqueror Index

Evaluate conquering adversity with the Adversity Conqueror Index ($ACI$):

$$ACI = \frac{\text{Effectiveness in conquering adversities}}{\text{Total instances of adversity conquering}}$$

### 8.4.6　Decision Boldness

Assess decision-making boldness with the Decision Boldness ($DB$):

$$DB = \frac{\text{Boldness displayed in decision-making}}{\text{Total instances of decision-making boldness}}$$

### 8.4.7　Empowerment Through Courage

Measure empowerment with the Courage Empowerment ($CE$):

$$CE = \frac{\text{Empowerment impact through displaying courage}}{\text{Total instances of empowerment in the story}}$$

Celebrate courage through the Courage Quotient, Fear Confrontation Index, Bold Action Score, Inspiration Cascade, Adversity Conqueror Index, Decision Boldness, and Courage Empowerment.

## 8.5　Connecting Through Shared Experiences

Forge connections through shared experiences with real and practical metrics capturing the essence of inspiring stories.

### 8.5.1　Connection Impact Score

Quantify connection impact with the Connection Impact Score ($CIS$):

$$CIS = \frac{\text{Impact of shared experiences on building connections}}{\text{Total instances of shared experiences}}$$

### 8.5.2　Empathy Quotient

Measure empathy with the Empathy Quotient ($EQ$):

$$EQ = \frac{\text{Empathy conveyed through shared experiences}}{\text{Total instances of empathy in the story}}$$

### 8.5.3 Common Struggle Unity Index

Assess unity through common struggles with the Common Struggle Unity Index ($CSUI$):

$$CSUI = \frac{\text{Unity fostered through common struggles}}{\text{Total instances of common struggles}}$$

### 8.5.4 Inspiration Network

Quantify inspiration with the Inspiration Network ($IN$):

$$IN = \frac{\text{Network effect of shared experiences on inspiring others}}{\text{Total instances of inspiration in the story}}$$

### 8.5.5 Triumph Together Index

Evaluate the power to triumph together with the Triumph Together Index ($TTI$):

$$TTI = \frac{\text{Effectiveness in overcoming challenges together}}{\text{Total instances of triumphing together}}$$

### 8.5.6 Decision Synergy

Assess decision-making synergy with the Decision Synergy ($DS$):

$$DS = \frac{\text{Synergy displayed in shared decision-making}}{\text{Total instances of decision-making synergy}}$$

### 8.5.7 Empowerment Through Connection

Measure empowerment with the Connection Empowerment ($CE$):

$$CE = \frac{\text{Empowerment impact through shared connections}}{\text{Total instances of empowerment in the story}}$$

Forge connections through shared experiences using the Connection Impact Score, Empathy Quotient, Common Struggle Unity Index, Inspiration Network, Triumph Together Index, Decision Synergy, and Connection Empowerment.

## 8.6 Honoring the Warrior Spirit

Celebrate the warrior spirit through real and practical metrics capturing the essence of inspiring stories.

### 8.6.1 Warrior Spirit Index

Quantify the warrior spirit with the Warrior Spirit Index ($WSI$):

$$WSI = \frac{\text{Overall warrior spirit displayed in the story}}{\text{Total instances of warrior spirit exhibited}}$$

### 8.6.2 Endurance Quotient

Measure endurance with the Endurance Quotient ($EQ$):

$$EQ = \frac{\text{Endurance demonstrated in facing challenges}}{\text{Total instances of endurance in the story}}$$

### 8.6.3 Fearless Action Score

Assess fearless actions with the Fearless Action Score ($FAS$):

$$FAS = \frac{\text{Impact of fearless actions on overcoming challenges}}{\text{Total instances of fearless actions}}$$

### 8.6.4 Inspiration Vanguard

Quantify inspiration with the Inspiration Vanguard ($IV$):

$$IV = \frac{\text{Vanguard effect of warrior spirit on inspiring others}}{\text{Total instances of inspiration in the story}}$$

### 8.6.5 Triumph Triumphantly Index

Evaluate triumphant triumphs with the Triumph Triumphantly Index ($TTI$):

$$TTI = \frac{\text{Effectiveness in triumphing triumphantly}}{\text{Total instances of triumphing triumphantly}}$$

### 8.6.6 Decision Valor

Assess decision-making valor with the Decision Valor ($DV$):

$$DV = \frac{\text{Valor displayed in decision-making}}{\text{Total instances of decision-making valor}}$$

### 8.6.7 Empowerment Through Warrior Spirit

Measure empowerment with the Warrior Spirit Empowerment ($WSE$):

$$WSE = \frac{\text{Empowerment impact through displaying the warrior spirit}}{\text{Total instances of empowerment in the story}}$$

Celebrate the warrior spirit through the Warrior Spirit Index, Endurance Quotient, Fearless Action Score, Inspiration Vanguard, Triumph Triumphantly Index, Decision Valor, and Warrior Spirit Empowerment.

## 8.7  A Tapestry of Triumphs

Explore a vibrant tapestry of triumphs through real and practical metrics capturing the essence of inspiring stories.

### 8.7.1  Tapestry Impact Score

Quantify the impact of the triumphs with the Tapestry Impact Score ($TIS$):

$$TIS = \frac{\text{Overall impact of triumphs displayed in the story}}{\text{Total instances of triumphs exhibited}}$$

### 8.7.2  Resilience Harmony Quotient

Measure harmony in resilience with the Resilience Harmony Quotient ($RHQ$):

$$RHQ = \frac{\text{Harmony displayed in resilience}}{\text{Total instances of resilience in the story}}$$

### 8.7.3  Inspiration Mosaic

Quantify inspiration with the Inspiration Mosaic ($IM$):

$$IM = \frac{\text{Mosaic effect of triumphs on inspiring others}}{\text{Total instances of inspiration in the story}}$$

### 8.7.4  Unity Through Triumph Index

Evaluate unity through triumphs with the Unity Through Triumph Index ($UTTI$):

$$UTTI = \frac{\text{Effectiveness in fostering unity through triumphs}}{\text{Total instances of unity through triumphs}}$$

### 8.7.5  Triumphal Decision-Making

Assess triumphal decision-making with the Triumphal Decision-Making ($TDM$):

$$TDM = \frac{\text{Triumph displayed in decision-making}}{\text{Total instances of triumphal decision-making}}$$

### 8.7.6 Empowerment Tapestry

Measure empowerment with the Tapestry Empowerment ($TE$):

$$TE = \frac{\text{Empowerment impact through the tapestry of triumphs}}{\text{Total instances of empowerment in the story}}$$

Explore the vibrant tapestry of triumphs through the Tapestry Impact Score, Resilience Harmony Quotient, Inspiration Mosaic, Unity Through Triumph Index, Triumphal Decision-Making, and Tapestry Empowerment.

# Chapter 9

# Research and Innovation

## 9.1 Advancements in Cancer Research

Explore the cutting-edge landscape of cancer research through real and practical metrics.

### 9.1.1 Research Impact Index

Quantify the impact of research with the Research Impact Index ($RII$):

$$RII = \frac{\text{Overall impact of cancer research}}{\text{Total instances of impactful research}}$$

### 9.1.2 Innovation Velocity

Measure the velocity of innovation with the Innovation Velocity ($IV$):

$$IV = \frac{\text{Speed of innovation in cancer research}}{\text{Total instances of innovative breakthroughs}}$$

### 9.1.3 Discovery Prowess

Quantify discovery prowess with the Discovery Prowess ($DP$):

$$DP = \frac{\text{Prowess in discovering new aspects of cancer}}{\text{Total instances of significant discoveries}}$$

### 9.1.4　Research Synergy Index

Evaluate synergy in research with the Research Synergy Index ($RSI$):

$$RSI = \frac{\text{Synergistic collaboration in cancer research}}{\text{Total instances of collaborative research}}$$

### 9.1.5　Innovative Treatment Efficacy

Assess treatment efficacy with Innovative Treatment Efficacy ($ITE$):

$$ITE = \frac{\text{Effectiveness of innovative treatments}}{\text{Total instances of successful innovative treatments}}$$

### 9.1.6　Data-driven Breakthroughs

Explore data-driven breakthroughs with the Data-driven Breakthroughs ($DB$):

$$DB = \frac{\text{Breakthroughs fueled by data-driven approaches}}{\text{Total instances of data-driven breakthroughs}}$$

### 9.1.7　Innovation Empowerment

Measure empowerment with the Innovation Empowerment ($IE$):

$$IE = \frac{\text{Empowerment impact through research and innovation}}{\text{Total instances of empowerment in cancer research}}$$

Delve into the forefront of cancer research with the Research Impact Index, Innovation Velocity, Discovery Prowess, Research Synergy Index, Innovative Treatment Efficacy, Data-driven Breakthroughs, and Innovation Empowerment.

## 9.2　Clinical Trials and Their Impact

Dive into the world of clinical trials and their impactful contributions through real and practical metrics.

### 9.2.1　Trial Effectiveness Score

Quantify the effectiveness of clinical trials with the Trial Effectiveness Score ($TES$):

$$TES = \frac{\text{Overall effectiveness of clinical trials}}{\text{Total instances of effective trials}}$$

### 9.2.2  Innovative Approaches Quotient

Measure innovation in trial approaches with the Innovative Approaches Quotient ($IAQ$):

$$IAQ = \frac{\text{Degree of innovation in trial methodologies}}{\text{Total instances of innovative trial approaches}}$$

### 9.2.3  Patient Impact Index

Quantify the impact on patients with the Patient Impact Index ($PII$):

$$PII = \frac{\text{Overall impact on patients from clinical trials}}{\text{Total instances of significant patient impact}}$$

### 9.2.4  Trial Diversity Dynamics

Evaluate diversity in trial participants with the Trial Diversity Dynamics ($TDD$):

$$TDD = \frac{\text{Dynamic representation in trial participants}}{\text{Total instances of diverse trial populations}}$$

### 9.2.5  Inclusive Trial Design

Assess inclusivity in trial design with the Inclusive Trial Design ($ITD$):

$$ITD = \frac{\text{Effectiveness of including diverse demographics in trial design}}{\text{Total instances of inclusive trial designs}}$$

### 9.2.6  Data-driven Precision Trials

Explore precision in trials with Data-driven Precision Trials ($DPT$):

$$DPT = \frac{\text{Precision achieved through data-driven trial approaches}}{\text{Total instances of precision trials}}$$

### 9.2.7  Patient Empowerment Through Trials

Measure patient empowerment with Patient Empowerment Through Trials ($PET$):

$$PET = \frac{\text{Empowerment impact on patients through clinical trials}}{\text{Total instances of patient empowerment in trials}}$$

Delve into the realm of clinical trials and their impact with the Trial Effectiveness Score, Innovative Approaches Quotient, Patient Impact Index, Trial Diversity Dynamics, Inclusive Trial Design, Data-driven Precision Trials, and Patient Empowerment Through Trials.

## 9.3 Genomic Medicine

Embark on the frontier of genomic medicine with real and practical insights presented in an accessible manner.

### 9.3.1 Genomic Precision Quotient

Quantify precision in genomic medicine with the Genomic Precision Quotient ($GPQ$):

$$GPQ = \frac{\text{Precision achieved through genomic medicine}}{\text{Total instances of precision in genomic interventions}}$$

### 9.3.2 Innovative Therapeutic Approaches

Explore innovation in therapeutic approaches with Innovative Therapeutic Approaches ($ITA$):

$$ITA = \frac{\text{Degree of innovation in genomic therapeutic methods}}{\text{Total instances of innovative genomic therapies}}$$

### 9.3.3 Genetic Marker Impact

Measure the impact of genetic markers with the Genetic Marker Impact ($GMI$):

$$GMI = \frac{\text{Overall impact of genetic markers in medical interventions}}{\text{Total instances of significant genetic marker impact}}$$

### 9.3.4 Genomic Diversity Dynamics

Evaluate diversity in genomic data with Genomic Diversity Dynamics ($GDD$):

$$GDD = \frac{\text{Dynamic representation in genomic data}}{\text{Total instances of diverse genomic data}}$$

### 9.3.5 Precision Diagnosis Index

Assess precision in diagnosis with the Precision Diagnosis Index ($PDI$):

$$PDI = \frac{\text{Effectiveness of precision diagnosis through genomic insights}}{\text{Total instances of precision diagnoses}}$$

### 9.3.6 Data-driven Genomic Insights

Explore data-driven insights with Data-driven Genomic Insights ($DGI$):

$$DGI = \frac{\text{Insights derived from data-driven genomic analyses}}{\text{Total instances of data-driven genomic insights}}$$

### 9.3.7 Patient Empowerment in Genomic Medicine

Measure patient empowerment with Patient Empowerment in Genomic Medicine ($PEG$):

$$PEG = \frac{\text{Empowerment impact on patients through genomic medicine}}{\text{Total instances of patient empowerment in genomic interventions}}$$

Embark on the frontier of genomic medicine with the Genomic Precision Quotient, Innovative Therapeutic Approaches, Genetic Marker Impact, Genomic Diversity Dynamics, Precision Diagnosis Index, Data-driven Genomic Insights, and Patient Empowerment in Genomic Medicine.

## 9.4 Immunotherapy Breakthroughs

Embark on a journey through impactful and practical insights into the realm of immunotherapy breakthroughs.

### 9.4.1 Immunotherapy Success Quotient

Quantify success in immunotherapy with the Immunotherapy Success Quotient ($ISQ$):

$$ISQ = \frac{\text{Success achieved through immunotherapy interventions}}{\text{Total instances of successful immunotherapies}}$$

### 9.4.2 Innovative Immunomodulation Strategies

Explore innovation in immunomodulation with Innovative Immunomodulation Strategies ($IIS$):

$$IIS = \frac{\text{Degree of innovation in immunomodulation methods}}{\text{Total instances of innovative immunomodulation strategies}}$$

### 9.4.3 Immune Response Impact

Measure the impact of immune responses with the Immune Response Impact ($IRI$):

$$IRI = \frac{\text{Overall impact of immune responses in medical interventions}}{\text{Total instances of significant immune response impact}}$$

### 9.4.4 Immunotherapy Diversity Dynamics

Evaluate diversity in immunotherapy approaches with Immunotherapy Diversity Dynamics ($IDD$):

$$IDD = \frac{\text{Dynamic representation in immunotherapy approaches}}{\text{Total instances of diverse immunotherapy methods}}$$

### 9.4.5 Precision Immunotherapy Index

Assess precision in immunotherapy with the Precision Immunotherapy Index ($PII$):

$$PII = \frac{\text{Effectiveness of precision immunotherapy approaches}}{\text{Total instances of precision immunotherapies}}$$

### 9.4.6 Data-driven Immunotherapy Insights

Explore data-driven insights with Data-driven Immunotherapy Insights ($DII$):

$$DII = \frac{\text{Insights derived from data-driven immunotherapy analyses}}{\text{Total instances of data-driven immunotherapy insights}}$$

### 9.4.7 Patient Empowerment Through Immunotherapy

Measure patient empowerment with Patient Empowerment Through Immunotherapy ($PETI$):

$$PETI = \frac{\text{Empowerment impact on patients through immunotherapy}}{\text{Total instances of patient empowerment in immunotherapies}}$$

Embark on a journey through immunotherapy breakthroughs with the Immunotherapy Success Quotient, Innovative Immunomodulation Strategies, Immune Response Impact, Immunotherapy Diversity Dynamics, Precision Immunotherapy Index, Data-driven Immunotherapy Insights, and Patient Empowerment Through Immunotherapy.

## 9.5 Future Trends in Cancer Treatment

Explore the future of cancer treatment through accessible and practical insights.

### 9.5.1 Treatment Evolution Quotient

Quantify the evolution of cancer treatment with the Treatment Evolution Quotient ($TEQ$):

$$TEQ = \frac{\text{Evolutionary progress in cancer treatment}}{\text{Total instances of evolved treatment methods}}$$

### 9.5.2 Innovative Therapeutic Modalities

Explore innovation in therapeutic modalities with Innovative Therapeutic Modalities ($ITM$):

$$ITM = \frac{\text{Degree of innovation in cancer therapeutic methods}}{\text{Total instances of innovative therapeutic modalities}}$$

### 9.5.3 Technology Integration Impact

Measure the impact of technology integration with the Technology Integration Impact ($TII$):

$$TII = \frac{\text{Overall impact of technology in cancer treatment}}{\text{Total instances of significant technology impact}}$$

### 9.5.4 Treatment Diversity Dynamics

Evaluate diversity in cancer treatment approaches with Treatment Diversity Dynamics ($TDD$):

$$TDD = \frac{\text{Dynamic representation in cancer treatment approaches}}{\text{Total instances of diverse treatment methods}}$$

### 9.5.5 Precision Treatment Index

Assess precision in cancer treatment with the Precision Treatment Index ($PTI$):

$$PTI = \frac{\text{Effectiveness of precision treatment approaches}}{\text{Total instances of precision cancer treatments}}$$

### 9.5.6 Data-driven Treatment Insights

Explore data-driven insights with Data-driven Treatment Insights ($DTI$):

$$DTI = \frac{\text{Insights derived from data-driven treatment analyses}}{\text{Total instances of data-driven treatment insights}}$$

### 9.5.7 Patient-Centric Future Trends

Anticipate patient-centric trends with Patient-Centric Future Trends ($PCFT$):

$$PCFT = \frac{\text{Adoption and impact of patient-centric trends in cancer treatment}}{\text{Total instances of patient-centric treatment trends}}$$

Embark on the journey of future trends in cancer treatment with the Treatment Evolution Quotient, Innovative Therapeutic Modalities, Technology Integration Impact, Treatment Diversity Dynamics, Precision Treatment Index, Data-driven Treatment Insights, and Patient-Centric Future Trends.

## 9.6 Patient Advocacy in Research

Uncover the vital role of patient advocacy in driving research forward with practical and accessible insights.

### 9.6.1 Advocacy Impact Quotient

Quantify the impact of patient advocacy with the Advocacy Impact Quotient ($AIQ$):

$$AIQ = \frac{\text{Impact of patient advocacy on research outcomes}}{\text{Total instances of impactful patient advocacy}}$$

### 9.6.2 Innovative Advocacy Strategies

Explore innovation in advocacy strategies with Innovative Advocacy Strategies ($IAS$):

$$IAS = \frac{\text{Degree of innovation in patient advocacy methods}}{\text{Total instances of innovative advocacy strategies}}$$

### 9.6.3 Patient-Centered Research Impact

Measure the impact of patient-centered research with the Patient-Centered Research Impact ($PCRI$):

$$PCRI = \frac{\text{Overall impact of patient-centered research initiatives}}{\text{Total instances of significant patient-centered research impact}}$$

### 9.6.4 Advocacy Diversity Dynamics

Evaluate diversity in advocacy approaches with Advocacy Diversity Dynamics ($ADD$):

$$ADD = \frac{\text{Dynamic representation in patient advocacy approaches}}{\text{Total instances of diverse advocacy methods}}$$

### 9.6.5 Precision Advocacy Index

Assess precision in advocacy with the Precision Advocacy Index ($PAI$):

$$PAI = \frac{\text{Effectiveness of precision advocacy approaches}}{\text{Total instances of precision advocacy initiatives}}$$

### 9.6.6 Data-driven Advocacy Insights

Explore data-driven insights with Data-driven Advocacy Insights ($DAI$):

$$DAI = \frac{\text{Insights derived from data-driven advocacy analyses}}{\text{Total instances of data-driven advocacy insights}}$$

### 9.6.7 Empowering Through Advocacy

Empower through advocacy with the Empowering Through Advocacy ($ETA$):

$$ETA = \frac{\text{Empowerment impact on patients through advocacy efforts}}{\text{Total instances of patient empowerment through advocacy}}$$

Uncover the vital role of patient advocacy in research with the Advocacy Impact Quotient, Innovative Advocacy Strategies, Patient-Centered Research Impact, Advocacy Diversity Dynamics, Precision Advocacy Index, Data-driven Advocacy Insights, and Empowering Through Advocacy.

## 9.7 Promoting Access to Innovative Therapies

Explore strategies for promoting access to innovative therapies in a simple and memorable way, incorporating real and practical insights.

### 9.7.1 Access Index

Quantify access to innovative therapies with the Access Index ($AI$):

$$AI = \frac{\text{Level of access to innovative therapies}}{\text{Total instances of improved access initiatives}}$$

### 9.7.2 Innovative Access Programs

Explore innovation in access programs with Innovative Access Programs ($IAP$):

$$IAP = \frac{\text{Degree of innovation in therapy access programs}}{\text{Total instances of innovative access programs}}$$

### 9.7.3 Patient-Centric Access

Prioritize patient-centric access with the Patient-Centric Access ($PCA$):

$$PCA = \frac{\text{Overall impact on patients through patient-centric access initiatives}}{\text{Total instances of patient-centric access impact}}$$

### 9.7.4 Access Diversity Dynamics

Evaluate diversity in access approaches with Access Diversity Dynamics ($ADD$):

$$ADD = \frac{\text{Dynamic representation in therapy access approaches}}{\text{Total instances of diverse access methods}}$$

### 9.7.5 Precision Access Index

Assess precision in therapy access with the Precision Access Index ($PAI$):

$$PAI = \frac{\text{Effectiveness of precision access approaches}}{\text{Total instances of precision access initiatives}}$$

### 9.7.6 Data-driven Access Insights

Explore data-driven insights with Data-driven Access Insights ($DAI$):

$$DAI = \frac{\text{Insights derived from data-driven access analyses}}{\text{Total instances of data-driven access insights}}$$

### 9.7.7 Community Engagement for Access

Engage communities for access with the Community Engagement for Access ($CEA$):

$$CEA = \frac{\text{Impact on therapy access through community engagement}}{\text{Total instances of community engagement for access}}$$

Discover strategies for promoting access to innovative therapies with the Access Index, Innovative Access Programs, Patient-Centric Access, Access Diversity Dynamics, Precision Access Index, Data-driven Access Insights, and Community Engagement for Access.

# Chapter 10

# Global Impact of Hope

## 10.1 Addressing Disparities in Cancer Care

Tackle disparities in cancer care with practical and memorable insights, emphasizing real-world solutions.

### 10.1.1 Disparities Reduction Quotient

Quantify efforts to reduce disparities with the Disparities Reduction Quotient ($DRQ$):

$$DRQ = \frac{\text{Reduction in cancer care disparities}}{\text{Total instances of successful disparities reduction efforts}}$$

### 10.1.2 Innovative Equity Initiatives

Explore innovation in equity initiatives with Innovative Equity Initiatives ($IEI$):

$$IEI = \frac{\text{Degree of innovation in cancer care equity programs}}{\text{Total instances of innovative equity initiatives}}$$

### 10.1.3 Patient-Centric Equity

Prioritize patient-centric equity with the Patient-Centric Equity ($PCE$):

$$PCE = \frac{\text{Overall impact on patients through patient-centric equity efforts}}{\text{Total instances of patient-centric equity impact}}$$

### 10.1.4   Equity Diversity Dynamics

Evaluate diversity in equity approaches with Equity Diversity Dynamics ($EDD$):

$$EDD = \frac{\text{Dynamic representation in cancer care equity approaches}}{\text{Total instances of diverse equity methods}}$$

### 10.1.5   Precision Equity Index

Assess precision in equity initiatives with the Precision Equity Index ($PEI$):

$$PEI = \frac{\text{Effectiveness of precision equity approaches}}{\text{Total instances of precision equity initiatives}}$$

### 10.1.6   Data-driven Equity Insights

Explore data-driven insights with Data-driven Equity Insights ($DEI$):

$$DEI = \frac{\text{Insights derived from data-driven equity analyses}}{\text{Total instances of data-driven equity insights}}$$

### 10.1.7   Community Collaboration for Equity

Foster community collaboration for equity with the Community Collaboration for Equity ($CCE$):

$$CCE = \frac{\text{Impact on equity through community collaboration}}{\text{Total instances of community collaboration for equity}}$$

Address disparities in cancer care with the Disparities Reduction Quotient, Innovative Equity Initiatives, Patient-Centric Equity, Equity Diversity Dynamics, Precision Equity Index, Data-driven Equity Insights, and Community Collaboration for Equity.

## 10.2   International Collaborations

Explore the power of international collaborations in cancer care with real-world insights and practical strategies.

### 10.2.1   Collaboration Effectiveness Index

Measure the effectiveness of collaborations with the Collaboration Effectiveness Index ($CEI$):

$$CEI = \frac{\text{Effectiveness of international collaborations in cancer care}}{\text{Total instances of successful collaboration efforts}}$$

### 10.2.2 Innovative Collaboration Models

Discover innovation in collaboration models with Innovative Collaboration Models ($ICM$):

$$ICM = \frac{\text{Degree of innovation in international cancer care collaboration models}}{\text{Total instances of innovative collaboration models}}$$

### 10.2.3 Patient-Centric Collaborations

Prioritize patient-centric collaborations with the Patient-Centric Collaborations ($PCC$):

$$PCC = \frac{\text{Overall impact on patients through patient-centric collaboration efforts}}{\text{Total instances of patient-centric collaboration impact}}$$

### 10.2.4 Collaboration Diversity Dynamics

Evaluate diversity in collaboration approaches with Collaboration Diversity Dynamics ($CDD$):

$$CDD = \frac{\text{Dynamic representation in international cancer care collaboration approaches}}{\text{Total instances of diverse collaboration methods}}$$

### 10.2.5 Precision Collaboration Index

Assess precision in collaboration initiatives with the Precision Collaboration Index ($PCI$):

$$PCI = \frac{\text{Effectiveness of precision collaboration approaches}}{\text{Total instances of precision collaboration initiatives}}$$

### 10.2.6 Data-driven Collaboration Insights

Explore data-driven insights with Data-driven Collaboration Insights ($DCI$):

$$DCI = \frac{\text{Insights derived from data-driven collaboration analyses}}{\text{Total instances of data-driven collaboration insights}}$$

### 10.2.7 Community Engagement in Collaboration

Enhance community engagement in collaboration with Community Engagement in Collaboration ($CEC$):

$$CEC = \frac{\text{Impact on collaboration through community engagement}}{\text{Total instances of community engagement in collaboration}}$$

Unleash the potential of international collaborations in cancer care with the Collaboration Effectiveness Index, Innovative Collaboration Models, Patient-Centric Collaborations, Collaboration Diversity Dynamics, Precision Collaboration Index, Data-driven Collaboration Insights, and Community Engagement in Collaboration.

## 10.3　Cancer Prevention on a Global Scale

Unlock the potential of global cancer prevention with actionable insights and practical approaches.

### 10.3.1　Prevention Effectiveness Quotient

Quantify the effectiveness of prevention strategies with the Prevention Effectiveness Quotient ($PEQ$):

$$PEQ = \frac{\text{Effectiveness of global cancer prevention efforts}}{\text{Total instances of successful prevention strategies}}$$

### 10.3.2　Innovative Prevention Models

Explore innovation in prevention models with Innovative Prevention Models ($IPM$):

$$IPM = \frac{\text{Degree of innovation in global cancer prevention models}}{\text{Total instances of innovative prevention models}}$$

### 10.3.3　Community-Centric Prevention

Prioritize community-centric prevention with the Community-Centric Prevention ($CCP$):

$$CCP = \frac{\text{Overall impact on communities through community-centric prevention efforts}}{\text{Total instances of community-centric prevention impact}}$$

### 10.3.4　Prevention Diversity Dynamics

Evaluate diversity in prevention approaches with Prevention Diversity Dynamics ($PDD$):

$$PDD = \frac{\text{Dynamic representation in global cancer prevention approaches}}{\text{Total instances of diverse prevention methods}}$$

### 10.3.5　Precision Prevention Index

Assess precision in prevention initiatives with the Precision Prevention Index ($PPI$):

$$PPI = \frac{\text{Effectiveness of precision prevention approaches}}{\text{Total instances of precision prevention initiatives}}$$

### 10.3.6　Data-driven Prevention Insights

Explore data-driven insights with Data-driven Prevention Insights ($DPI$):

$$DPI = \frac{\text{Insights derived from data-driven prevention analyses}}{\text{Total instances of data-driven prevention insights}}$$

### 10.3.7 International Collaboration in Prevention

Strengthen international collaboration in prevention with International Collaboration in Prevention ($ICP$):

$$ICP = \frac{\text{Impact on prevention through global collaboration}}{\text{Total instances of international collaboration in prevention}}$$

Take charge of global cancer prevention with the Prevention Effectiveness Quotient, Innovative Prevention Models, Community-Centric Prevention, Prevention Diversity Dynamics, Precision Prevention Index, Data-driven Prevention Insights, and International Collaboration in Prevention.

## 10.4 Innovative Programs Around the World

Embark on a journey of transformative global programs addressing cancer challenges with real-world insights and practical approaches.

### 10.4.1 Program Impact Quotient

Measure the impact of global programs with the Program Impact Quotient ($PIQ$):

$$PIQ = \frac{\text{Overall impact of innovative global programs}}{\text{Total instances of successful program implementations}}$$

### 10.4.2 Trailblazing Program Models

Explore trailblazing program models with Trailblazing Program Models ($TPM$):

$$TPM = \frac{\text{Degree of innovation in global cancer program models}}{\text{Total instances of innovative program models}}$$

### 10.4.3 Community-Centered Program Development

Prioritize community-centered program development with Community-Centered Program Development ($CCPD$):

$$CCPD = \frac{\text{Overall impact on communities through community-centered program efforts}}{\text{Total instances of community-centered program impact}}$$

### 10.4.4 Program Diversity Dynamics

Evaluate diversity in program approaches with Program Diversity Dynamics ($PDD$):

$$PDD = \frac{\text{Dynamic representation in global cancer program approaches}}{\text{Total instances of diverse program methods}}$$

### 10.4.5 Precision Program Index

Assess precision in program initiatives with the Precision Program Index ($PPI$):

$$PPI = \frac{\text{Effectiveness of precision program approaches}}{\text{Total instances of precision program initiatives}}$$

### 10.4.6 Data-driven Program Insights

Explore data-driven insights with Data-driven Program Insights ($DPI$):

$$DPI = \frac{\text{Insights derived from data-driven program analyses}}{\text{Total instances of data-driven program insights}}$$

### 10.4.7 Global Collaboration in Program Development

Strengthen global collaboration in program development with Global Collaboration in Program Development ($GCPD$):

$$GCPD = \frac{\text{Impact on program development through global collaboration}}{\text{Total instances of international collaboration in program development}}$$

Embark on a global journey of cancer solutions with the Program Impact Quotient, Trailblazing Program Models, Community-Centered Program Development, Program Diversity Dynamics, Precision Program Index, Data-driven Program Insights, and Global Collaboration in Program Development.

## 10.5 Cultural Perspectives on Healing

Uncover the rich tapestry of global healing through diverse cultural perspectives with real-world insights and practical considerations.

### 10.5.1 Cultural Healing Quotient

Explore the impact of cultural perspectives on healing with the Cultural Healing Quotient ($CHQ$):

$$CHQ = \frac{\text{Overall impact of cultural healing perspectives}}{\text{Total instances of successful cultural healing practices}}$$

### 10.5.2 Harmony in Healing Traditions

Discover harmony in healing traditions with Harmony in Healing Traditions ($HHT$):

$$HHT = \frac{\text{Degree of harmony in global cultural healing traditions}}{\text{Total instances of harmonious healing practices}}$$

### 10.5.3  Community-Centric Healing Approaches

Embrace community-centric healing with Community-Centric Healing Approaches ($CCHA$):

$$CCHA = \frac{\text{Overall impact on communities through community-centric healing efforts}}{\text{Total instances of community-centric healing impact}}$$

### 10.5.4  Healing Diversity Dynamics

Appreciate diversity in healing approaches with Healing Diversity Dynamics ($HDD$):

$$HDD = \frac{\text{Dynamic representation in global healing approaches}}{\text{Total instances of diverse healing methods}}$$

### 10.5.5  Precision Healing Index

Assess precision in healing initiatives with the Precision Healing Index ($PHI$):

$$PHI = \frac{\text{Effectiveness of precision healing approaches}}{\text{Total instances of precision healing initiatives}}$$

### 10.5.6  Data-driven Healing Insights

Unearth data-driven insights with Data-driven Healing Insights ($DHI$):

$$DHI = \frac{\text{Insights derived from data-driven healing analyses}}{\text{Total instances of data-driven healing insights}}$$

### 10.5.7  Cross-Cultural Collaboration in Healing

Foster cross-cultural collaboration in healing with Cross-Cultural Collaboration in Healing ($CCCH$):

$$CCCH = \frac{\text{Impact on healing through cross-cultural collaboration}}{\text{Total instances of international collaboration in healing}}$$

Embark on a global journey of healing traditions with the Cultural Healing Quotient, Harmony in Healing Traditions, Community-Centric Healing Approaches, Healing Diversity Dynamics, Precision Healing Index, Data-driven Healing Insights, and Cross-Cultural Collaboration in Healing.

## 10.6  Empowering Developing Nations

Explore innovative strategies to empower developing nations in their fight against cancer with real-world insights and practical considerations.

### 10.6.1 Health Equity Index

Evaluate health equity with the Health Equity Index ($HEI$):

$$HEI = \frac{\text{Equity in access to cancer care}}{\text{Total instances of health equity initiatives}}$$

### 10.6.2 Resource Mobilization Efficiency

Assess efficiency in resource mobilization with the Resource Mobilization Efficiency ($RME$):

$$RME = \frac{\text{Efficiency in mobilizing resources for cancer care}}{\text{Total instances of successful resource mobilization}}$$

### 10.6.3 Capacity Building Impact

Measure impact in capacity building with the Capacity Building Impact ($CBI$):

$$CBI = \frac{\text{Impact on healthcare capacity building}}{\text{Total instances of successful capacity building efforts}}$$

### 10.6.4 Technology Transfer Quotient

Facilitate technology transfer with the Technology Transfer Quotient ($TTQ$):

$$TTQ = \frac{\text{Successful transfer of medical technology}}{\text{Total instances of technology transfer initiatives}}$$

### 10.6.5 Sustainable Healthcare Development

Promote sustainable healthcare development with the Sustainable Healthcare Development ($SHD$):

$$SHD = \frac{\text{Sustainability of healthcare initiatives in developing nations}}{\text{Total instances of sustainable healthcare projects}}$$

### 10.6.6 Community Engagement Vitality

Enhance community engagement with the Community Engagement Vitality ($CEV$):

$$CEV = \frac{\text{Vitality of community engagement in healthcare}}{\text{Total instances of vibrant community involvement}}$$

### 10.6.7 Policy Advocacy Effectiveness

Evaluate policy advocacy with the Policy Advocacy Effectiveness ($PAE$):

$$PAE = \frac{\text{Effectiveness of cancer care policy advocacy}}{\text{Total instances of successful policy advocacy}}$$

Empower developing nations on their journey towards effective cancer care with the Health Equity Index, Resource Mobilization Efficiency, Capacity Building Impact, Technology Transfer Quotient, Sustainable Healthcare Development, Community Engagement Vitality, and Policy Advocacy Effectiveness.

## 10.7 Hope as a Universal Language

Explore the transformative power of hope as a universal language, transcending borders and bringing positive change to communities worldwide.

### 10.7.1 Hope Index Formula

Quantify the impact of hope with the Hope Index Formula ($HI$):

$$HI = \frac{\text{Magnitude of hope}}{\text{Total instances of hope-driven initiatives}}$$

### 10.7.2 Cross-Cultural Hope Synergy

Uncover the synergy of hope across cultures with Cross-Cultural Hope Synergy ($CCHS$):

$$CCHS = \frac{\text{Harmony in cross-cultural hope initiatives}}{\text{Total instances of cross-cultural hope synergy}}$$

### 10.7.3 Community Resilience Quotient

Measure community resilience with the Community Resilience Quotient ($CRQ$):

$$CRQ = \frac{\text{Strength of communities in the face of challenges}}{\text{Total instances of community resilience}}$$

### 10.7.4 Global Hope Dynamics

Analyze global hope dynamics with Global Hope Dynamics ($GHD$):

$$GHD = \frac{\text{Impact of hope on a global scale}}{\text{Total instances of global hope dynamics}}$$

### 10.7.5 Inclusive Hope Strategies

Promote inclusivity with Inclusive Hope Strategies ($IHS$):

$$IHS = \frac{\text{Effectiveness of inclusive hope strategies}}{\text{Total instances of inclusive hope initiatives}}$$

### 10.7.6 Hope Data Insights

Leverage data for insights with Hope Data Insights ($HDI$):

$$HDI = \frac{\text{Insights derived from data-driven hope analyses}}{\text{Total instances of hope-driven data insights}}$$

### 10.7.7 Cross-Border Hope Collaborations

Foster collaboration through borders with Cross-Border Hope Collaborations ($CBHC$):

$$CBHC = \frac{\text{Impact on hope through cross-border collaborations}}{\text{Total instances of international hope partnerships}}$$

Embark on a journey where hope serves as a universal language, connecting hearts and minds through the Hope Index Formula, Cross-Cultural Hope Synergy, Community Resilience Quotient, Global Hope Dynamics, Inclusive Hope Strategies, Hope Data Insights, and Cross-Border Hope Collaborations.

# Chapter 11

# Reflections on the Journey

## 11.1 Looking Back with Gratitude

Embark on a reflective journey, exploring the power of gratitude and its impact on personal well-being and resilience.

### 11.1.1 Gratitude Quotient (GQ)

Quantify the level of gratitude with the Gratitude Quotient ($GQ$):

$$GQ = \frac{\text{Total expressions of gratitude}}{\text{Duration of reflective period (in days)}}$$

### 11.1.2 Gratitude Journaling

Enhance well-being through Gratitude Journaling:

$$\text{Gratitude Score (GS)} = \frac{\text{Number of entries in gratitude journal}}{\text{Total reflections}}$$

### 11.1.3 Impact of Gratitude Practices

Evaluate the impact of gratitude practices:

$$\text{Impact Index (II)} = \frac{\text{Positive outcomes attributed to gratitude}}{\text{Total instances of gratitude practices}}$$

### 11.1.4 Gratitude Resilience Equation

Measure resilience through the Gratitude Resilience Equation ($GRE$):

$$GRE = \frac{\text{Resilience level post-reflection}}{\text{Initial resilience level}}$$

### 11.1.5 Expressing Gratitude Chemically

Explore the chemical expressions of gratitude:

$$\text{Chemical Formula for Gratitude} : C_8H_{11}NO_2S$$

### 11.1.6 Gratitude Frequency Spectrum

Analyze the frequency of gratitude expressions:

$$\text{Frequency Spectrum (FS)} = \frac{\text{Variety of gratitude expressions}}{\text{Total gratitude expressions}}$$

### 11.1.7 Gratitude Ripple Effect

Witness the ripple effect of gratitude:

$$\text{Ripple Magnitude (RM)} = \frac{\text{Positive impact on others}}{\text{Total instances of gratitude ripple}}$$

In this reflective journey, uncover the mathematical beauty of gratitude with the Gratitude Quotient, Gratitude Journaling, Impact of Gratitude Practices, Gratitude Resilience Equation, Chemical Expressions of Gratitude, Gratitude Frequency Spectrum, and Gratitude Ripple Effect.

## 11.2 Lessons Learned

Embark on a reflective journey, exploring profound lessons learned throughout the cancer journey, blending practical wisdom with mathematical insights.

### 11.2.1 Lessons in Resilience

Quantify the resilience gained through challenges:

$$\text{Resilience Quotient (RQ)} = \frac{\text{Total challenges faced}}{\text{Resilience level after overcoming challenges}}$$

### 11.2.2  Equation of Personal Growth

Express personal growth through an equation:

$$\text{Personal Growth Equation (PGE)} : \text{Growth} = \frac{\text{Knowledge gained}}{\text{Initial understanding}}$$

### 11.2.3  Graph of Emotional Waves

Visualize emotional fluctuations:

$$\text{Emotional Wave Amplitude (EWA)} = \frac{\text{Difference between emotional peaks and troughs}}{\text{Duration of emotional journey}}$$

### 11.2.4  Time-Value of Support

Quantify the impact of support over time:

$$\text{Support Value Over Time (SVOT)} = \frac{\text{Support received}}{\text{Total time in treatment}}$$

### 11.2.5  Energy Conservation Principle

Apply the energy conservation principle:

$$\text{Energy Conservation} : \text{Energy expended during challenges} = \text{Energy gained from overcoming challenges}$$

### 11.2.6  Lessons in Probability

Analyze the probability of positive outcomes:

$$\text{Probability of Positive Outcome (PPO)} = \frac{\text{Number of positive outcomes}}{\text{Total number of outcomes}}$$

### 11.2.7  Optimism Index

Evaluate the level of optimism attained:

$$\text{Optimism Index (OI)} = \frac{\text{Optimistic outlook score}}{\text{Initial outlook score}}$$

In this exploration of lessons learned, delve into the mathematical tapestry woven into the fabric of personal growth, resilience, emotional dynamics, support dynamics, energy conservation, probability, and optimism.

## 11.3　Expressing Personal Growth

Embark on a numerical exploration of personal growth, blending real-world insights with mathematical formulas.

### 11.3.1　Quantifying Knowledge Gain

Measure the knowledge gained during the journey:

$$\text{Knowledge Gain} = \text{Final knowledge level} - \text{Initial knowledge level}$$

### 11.3.2　Rate of Personal Growth

Calculate the rate of personal growth:

$$\text{Rate of Growth} = \frac{\text{Knowledge Gain}}{\text{Time elapsed}}$$

### 11.3.3　The Growth Function

Model personal growth as a function of time:

$$\text{Growth}(t) = \frac{\text{Knowledge Gain}}{\text{Time elapsed}} \times t$$

### 11.3.4　Embracing Change Equation

Express the positive impact of embracing change:

$$\text{Embracing Change Index (ECI)} = \frac{\text{Positive changes embraced}}{\text{Total changes encountered}}$$

### 11.3.5　Resilience as a Growth Factor

Incorporate resilience into the growth equation:

$$\text{Total Growth} = \text{Rate of Growth} + \text{Resilience Bonus}$$

### 11.3.6　Graph of Personal Growth

Visualize the growth trajectory:

$$\text{Personal Growth Curve} : \text{Growth} = f(t)$$

Explore the synergy between personal experiences and mathematical expressions, quantifying the transformative journey of personal growth.

## 11.4 Honoring the Support System

Acknowledge the invaluable support system with a blend of heartfelt gratitude and mathematical symbolism.

### 11.4.1 Gratitude Equation

Express gratitude mathematically:

$$\text{Gratitude} = \sum_{i=1}^{n} \left( \frac{\text{Impact of Support from Person } i}{\text{Magnitude of Support from Person } i} \right)$$

### 11.4.2 Support Vector Calculation

Quantify the strength and direction of support:

$$\text{Support Vector} = \langle \text{Strength of Emotional Support}, \text{Strength of Practical Support} \rangle$$

### 11.4.3 Support Matrix Determinant

Measure the overall impact of the support matrix:

$$\text{Support Matrix} = \begin{vmatrix} \text{Emotional Support} & \text{Practical Support} \\ \text{Informational Support} & \text{Companionship} \end{vmatrix}$$

### 11.4.4 Resilience Coefficient

Factor in the resilience of the support system:

$$\text{Resilience Coefficient} = \frac{\text{Total Resilience of Support System}}{\text{Number of Supportive Individuals}}$$

### 11.4.5 Support Energy Theorem

Relate the support system to energy conservation:

$$\text{Support Energy} = \text{Potential Support} + \text{Kinetic Support}$$

### 11.4.6 Graph of Support Impact

Visualize the impact of the support system over time:

$$\text{Support Impact Curve} : \text{Impact} = f(\text{Time})$$

Capture the essence of gratitude and the mathematical harmony within the support system.

## 11.5 Moving Forward with Hope

Transition into the future with a blend of optimism and mathematical resonance.

### 11.5.1 Hopeful Equation

Define hope as a mathematical concept:

$$\text{Hope} = \frac{\text{Number of Possibilities}}{\text{Level of Optimism}}$$

### 11.5.2 Equation of Resilience

Quantify the ability to bounce back:

$$\text{Resilience} = \frac{\text{Total Challenges Overcome}}{\text{Personal Growth Factor}}$$

### 11.5.3 Hope Vector Calculation

Compute the direction and magnitude of hope:

$$\text{Hope Vector} = \langle \text{Direction of Dreams}, \text{Magnitude of Determination} \rangle$$

### 11.5.4 Equation of Moving Forward

Express the process of moving forward mathematically:

$$\text{Moving Forward} = \int_{\text{Present}}^{\text{Future}} \text{Optimism}(t)\, dt$$

### 11.5.5 Hope Function

Model hope as a function of time:

$$\text{Hope Function} : \text{Hope} = f(\text{Time})$$

### 11.5.6  Hopeful Constants

Identify the constants that contribute to sustained hope:

$$\text{Hope Constants} = \{\text{Faith}, \text{Persistence}, \text{Support}\}$$

Embrace the mathematical elegance of moving forward with hope.

## 11.6  Acknowledging Resilience

Celebrate the strength and perseverance with a touch of mathematical acknowledgment.

### 11.6.1  Resilience Quotient

Quantify the level of resilience using the Resilience Quotient:

$$\text{Resilience Quotient} = \frac{\text{Total Challenges Overcome}}{\text{Personal Growth Factor}}$$

### 11.6.2  Persistence Formula

Express the power of persistence as a formula:

$$\text{Persistence} = \frac{\text{Number of Attempts}}{\text{Obstacles Overcome}}$$

### 11.6.3  Strength-to-Challenge Ratio

Define the balance between strength and challenges:

$$\text{Strength-to-Challenge Ratio} = \frac{\text{Strength}}{\text{Challenges Faced}}$$

### 11.6.4  Resilience Wave Function

Model resilience as a dynamic wave:

$$\text{Resilience Wave Function} : \text{Resilience} = f(\text{Time})$$

### 11.6.5 Overcoming Adversity Matrix

Present a matrix depicting the process of overcoming adversity:

$$\begin{bmatrix} \text{Adversity}_1 & \text{Overcome}_1 \\ \text{Adversity}_2 & \text{Overcome}_2 \end{bmatrix}$$

Acknowledge resilience with the elegance of mathematical representation.

## 11.7 Epilogue: The Everlasting Formula for Hope

Conclude the journey with a symbolic formula capturing the essence of enduring hope.

### 11.7.1 Hope Equation

Express the everlasting nature of hope through the Hope Equation:

$$\text{Hope} = \frac{\text{Courage} \times \text{Faith}}{\text{Resilience}}$$

### 11.7.2 Perseverance Constant

Define the constant that signifies perpetual perseverance:

$$\text{Perseverance Constant} = e^{\pi i}$$

### 11.7.3 Infinity of Possibilities

Illustrate the infinity of possibilities with a mathematical expression:

$$\text{Possibilities} = \lim_{x \to \infty} \left( 1 + \frac{1}{x} \right)^x$$

### 11.7.4 Eternal Optimism

Capture the eternal aspect of optimism with a simple yet powerful equation:

$$\text{Optimism} = \frac{\text{Joy} \times \text{Belief}}{\text{Time}}$$

Conclude the journey with the poetic beauty of mathematical formulations, emphasizing the enduring nature of hope.

www.ingramcontent.com/pod-product-compliance
Lightning Source LLC
Chambersburg PA
CBHW082338270726
48658CB00017B/2890